D1488351

The 85% Solution
2nd Edition

WRITTEN & COPYRIGHT BY DAN PURSER MD

MTHFR is Overpowering Our Medical System - Chances Are You Have It Too...

WHAT'S COVERED IN THIS VERY DETAILED WORK:

- Methylation | MTHFR Mutation
- Folate Deficiency
- Methylfolate use
- MTHFR Homozygous | MTHFR C677T | MTHFR A1298C | MTHFR Heterozygous
- MTHFR Gene | MTHFR Testing
- Methylation Cycle | Methylation Analysis
- Methylfolate Trap | MTHFR Deficiency
- MTHFR Treatment Protocols detailed
- MTHFR Diet | MTHFR Support

MY LEGAL PROTECTION

THIS BOOK IS for educational information and entertainment purposes only. Please do not use the information contained in this book to treat yourself. Please consult with a knowledgeable physician in your area before starting any treatment as might possibly be suggested in this book. I will not be held responsible if something goes wrong. So BE CAREFUL!

Also, please get Dr. Ben Lynch's book – MTHFR BASICS – as he is clearly the pre-eminent knowledge on this subject, and I am just an M.D. trying to give it a more western medical twist.

Thank you.

CONTENTS

GO TO AUSTIMBOOKDOWNLOAD.STRIKINGLY.COM TO
DOWNLOAD YOUR FREE #1 BESTSELLING AUTISM BOOK AND
TO JOIN DR PURSER'S EMAIL LIST MORE FREE BOOKS AND
INFO!

SUCCESS! YOU MADE IT!
CHOOSE YOUR DOWNLOAD BELOW:

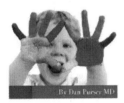

WELCOME TO MODERN MEDICINE -- YOU
HAVE A FAMILY MEMBER WITH ASD AND YOU
JUST KNOW THERE ARE SOME ANSWERS,
SOME HELP, SOME WHERE...

THERE IS...

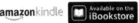

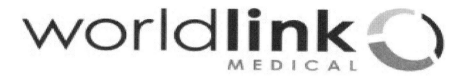

About Dan Purser MD

As just your plain old run-of-the-mill a physician, I was seeing a lot of confusion about hormones and preventive medicine. Heck, even I was confused (even the government was too, and is still confused to this day, but back then they had shoved the food pyramid down our throat and then decided to change it to it's newest iteration – what a mess!). I was also heavily involved in pituitary endocrinology research at a university level, plus held down a day job in a cosmetic surgery group where I dealt with complex wound and healing issues. So needing to be even more overwhelmed on a daily basis I decided to write a much needed textbook on preventive medicine. Small grew to huge and eventually we published my first book -- a 750-page ride into academic medicine. The book was a big hit at shows and conferences -- so I got a little inkling on how well books could do.

I spun off shorter versions of my textbook (Male/Female Handbook A & B). Then I wrote my first #1 book PROGESTERONE. I've written many books since, 11 more which have been #1 in various categories on Amazon.

And learned that books, even #1 books, make you little money. But the speaking gigs (now 5 figures minimum to speak), and product design and sales opportunities around twelve #1 books are AWESOME.

So I keep writing. I speak somewhere in the world (Hello Borneo!!!) at least once a month, we'll be manufacturing over 200 products this year (hint= TONS of $$$), and this year (2016) my goal is to teach physicians how to gain my lifestyle and success – there's tons of pie out there and I want to share it. Thanks and I love you all –

Dan Purser MD

FIND ALL OF DR PURSERS BOOKS HERE

greatmedebooks.com

Progesterone: http://goo.gl/yIAAWo

Testosterone: http://goo.gl/WiJiiC

Fibromyalgia: http://amzn.to/22Lt9iT

Breast Cancer: http://amzn.to/1RaEPaV

Osteoporosis: http://goo.gl/Dg9Atx

ED Book: http://amzn.to/1Z9QlrP

Healthy Menopause and Essential Oils: http://goo.gl/rqviCB

The 85% SOLUTION: http://goo.gl/dqSi9p

Natural Therapies for Autism: Updates on the Research:
http://goo.gl/CnfGry

FOREWORD

I'M A WESTERN M.D.

Kind of...

I have, in the last few years, started to wander far afield. I deal with complex wound and healing issues in a plastic surgery group in Utah – it's a VERY unique opportunity that I have for my day job. I've also done endocrinology research on the side at a major university hospital on the west coast, written more than a dozen books and published them on Amazon (including a textbook and TEN #1 books!), designed products for various vitamin companies, spoken all over the world, have a cash only practice and eschew the deafening control of insurance companies.

Yep, pretty far afield. But it may surprise you (it does me) that I have been one of my county's Utah Medical Association reps the last 11 years. What were they thinking?

But what was I *thinking* when I wrote this book? This problem has flummoxed me. I'm not even sure why I wrote this other than for myself. And then I realized...

What a problem it was.

Do you have or have ever had problems with addictions, smoking, drugs, alcohol, Down's syndrome, miscarriages, pulmonary emboli, depression, schizophrenia, fibromyalgia, chronic fatigue syndrome, chemical sensitivity, Parkinson's Disease, Irritable Bowel Syndrome, Pre-eclampsia? Or any other unexplained chronic diseases where the doctor just shook his head?

Have others in your family had any of these (or other diseases listed in Chapter Six)?

You can see why I think this is overwhelming – I keep tracing down so many illnesses linked to this problem. And these are patients who've been to a dozen or more other doctors. This IS overwhelming our healthcare system and is not being recognized (IMHO).

Have you ever had intracellular vitamin testing done? (Well, you will after this book.)

Why does your doctor (my brothers and sisters in the medical field who are REALLY WESTERN medical doctors) miss this? They have time for Bandaids® only – too busy with their 60+ patients and crushing schedule that makes them hate life. So you have to stop him short, grab her attention, whatever you can do. And hand them this book (on your iPad or paperback version) and if it's you (you'll know when you're done with it) then tell them it's you, and to read it and to help you. NOW.

Then see if they do…

Let's read through this together – because I wrote this for me – it was a complex subject which I was too busy to digest and too in a hurry to figure out. But if I know my talents, one that I ABSOLUTELY know that I have is to make the complex simple and understandable. So I hope this helps.

I have been involved in pituitary endocrinology research for years and writing about it (how ironic that I called it the great mimic – I was wrong – this is THE GREATEST MIMIC) – plus I see patients that are difficult to diagnose and treat at my practice in Lindon. I also perform SpectraCell™ Comprehensive MicroNutrient Panels on most of my patients (an amazing test that looks at INTRACELLULAR vitamin and mineral levels). And over the years I have seen tons of patient with B12 and folate levels that just would not correct – thus I backed into MTHFR.

This book is written for my patients and loved ones – a compilation really by people and other doctors who were forerunners in this field – I am just a reporter now. But I hope bringing it together and organizing it all under one title can help make it a little easier.

You'd better learn this diagram backwards and forward:

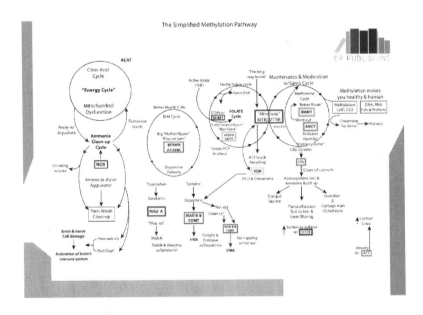

IT STARTS WITH A WOMAN...

She came into the Garden Room and sat down – she looked sad, aged beyond her years, too. When I walked in, her appearance made me glance at her chart.

I did the math - she was only 34.

Only 34...

I'd never seen her before, so I asked who referred her.

She said the name of another patient. "She said you were good – would take the time with me. I've been to 12 other doctors or something - lost count. Most of them didn't have a clue."

I nodded and looked at her papers and labs. I told her a little about me – researcher, author, physician, no more than eight patients in a day - that kinda stuff. It was an old song for me.

"So WHAT IS the matter with you?" I smiled a little around the edges. I looked at her straight in the eyes, weighing her. I already suspected.

She looked plainly back. "You tell me. Depressed, fatigued, EXHAUSTED ALL THE TIME."

I nodded. Made quick notes. I don't use an EMR – all my doc patients would shoot me first if I tried. They were NOT private and we all knew it. So I scribbled with a black pen.

"Cold hands and feet, ICE COLD. Hair loss. Periods are wack. I've had two kids, both C-section. Felt really bad for ten plus years."

I looked up.

"They've had me on everything – Cymbalta™, Prozac™, BCPs to regulate my period – made me worse. Adderall™, Provigil™ for the fatigue. Nothing worked..."

"Still taking anything?"

"Stopped it all – it made me worse."

"Your labs look like you're in ovarian failure maybe, certainly ovarian insufficiency."

"What's that?"

"Your ovaries have the dwindles." I smiled at her – sadly. I'd seen this before, but I was being careful.

"Yah, that's why they put me on birth control pills but those weirded me out." She leaned forward. "What's that mean – why aren't they working?"

"It doesn't look like pituitary problems – any head injuries?"

She shook her head.

"Were your deliveries crazy? Or loss of blood? Anything?"

"Both were Caeserean. And no bleeding or trauma other than the surgery. Easy."

I nodded and looked at her labs, thinking, pondering my next move.

"I just want to die most days. And I am so tired. My husband thinks I'm crazy."

"Anything like this in your family?"

"Had two aunts on my mom's side. A cousin, too. My sister has schizophrenia."

I nodded. She dug in her bag and pulled out a huge sheath of papers. "This is all my labs and medical reports." She slid them towards me and I reeled them in.

"Thanks, I'll definitely look at them."

"We've spent probably $18,000 dollars on all of this." She shook her head.

I nodded and leaned forward. "When did all this start?

"After high school – in college. And I've never recovered."

"Do any drugs or party?"

"Nah, went to Brigham Young University. Are you LDS?"

I nodded. My practice was in Lindon, Utah just a few miles from BYU. I went there, too.

"Were you a cheerleader or gymnast?"

She laughed, looked down at her body, then looked at me. "Really?

This was a lady on her last leg. She'd had it.

"I'll go through everything here," I touched the pile of reports. "Then you can pay me for this visit, but today why don't you pay me for another test instead." I dug through my box and set a copy of a SpectraCell™ Comprehensive Micronutrient Panel in front of her – it was one of my own results.

She looked at it.

"This test looks at intracellular vitamins and minerals – it will tell us a lot as to why your ovaries aren't working and as to why you're so tired."

She nodded.

"Let's spend your money on that test instead."

"Any promises it'll work for me?"

"None, and the test always works meaning it gives us great data, but no one else has ever done this on you, so you never know. My gut, and 27 years of practice tell me it's not your pituitary. And we use this in research – it will be really helpful and may give us a roadmap as to which way to go. It's also a root cause kind of thing."

She nodded, thinking. "Heard you look for root causes. Let's do it."

I smiled.

1

ROOT CAUSES OF THE MTHFR MUTATION

THE CURRENT HUMAN race lives and procreates a long time.

I had just had a daughter and was turning 50.

Wow, was I crazy or what?

It wasn't that long ago that the average American lived to be in their late 20's (three generations back), women were getting married in their teens and having babies, then dying in child birth. Only one out of ten children lived to adulthood – much lower in other countries. Now we're living into our 90's regularly. With our longer life expectancy, we are passing on more gene defects. There's no doubt. It's just the way it is.

MTHFR (ACTUALLY called MethyleneTetraHydroFolate Reductase Enzyme Deficiency) came along in northern Europe several hundred generations ago and now has blown up (85% of the population carries a variant or at least a SNP of this gene mutation[1] [stands for Single Nucleotide Polymorphism] or more appropriately called a transcription error, 5% carries both genes so are homozygous). And oddly enough 49% of the Latino or Hispanic population are carriers or have the MTHFR disease. Well, I guess it's not really a disease or mutation – it's actually just a DNA replication or copying problem called a TRANSCRIPTION ERROR. Wow, what an error.

Methylation is probably THE most important enzyme function our body makes – it controls so much – and is deeply and inherently tied to our energy levels, both perceived and actual.

You always have to wonder how mutations survive – especially cruddy ones like this one – studies have shown that it's a survival gene mutation against colon cancer[2] (crazy right? But I knew it had to give some type of x-man powers).

And why does your doctor not know about this or recognize it? I'm not sure. I think my brothers and sisters in the medical field are just too busy with getting patients out of the office – they are overwhelmed, seeing 60 patients a day (I never see more than 8).

This book, always a work in motion, makes an attempt at detailing the diagnosis, diseases, and treatments of this disease more thoroughly to make it all more comprehensible for you and me.

2

HERE'S WHAT A HEALTHY MTHFR GENE DOES FOR YOU

The breath-taking in scope Human Genome Project was completed in April of 2003. The Project's goal was to provide researchers with powerful tools to understand the genetic factors in human disease, paving the way for new strategies for their diagnosis, treatment and prevention[3] - this fueled the discovery of more than 1,800 disease genes including MTHFR problems (transcription errors). When it's all working right, the MTHFR genes, on Chromosome 1, begin a multi-step chemical methylation process, which goes like this:

➤ The MTHFR gene leads to production of the MTHFR enzyme.

➤ The MTHFR enzyme works with the folate vitamins (B9, folic acid), breaking it down from 5,10-methylenetetrahydrofolate to 5-methyltetrahydrofolate

➤ 5-methyltetrahydrofolate helps convert the amino acid homocysteine down to another essential amino acid, methionine, which is used by your body to make proteins, utilize antioxidants, and to assist your liver to process fats. Methionine helps with depression, reduces inflammation and helps convert estradiol (E2) into estriol (E3) (i.e. critical to hormone production – where I tend to come in).

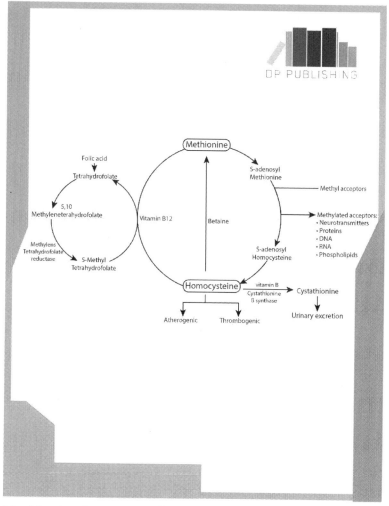

> Methionine is converted in your liver into SAM-e (s-adenosylmethionine), which is anti-inflammatory, supports your immune system, helps produce critical brain chemicals such as serotonin, dopamine and melatonin, and is involved in the growth, repair and maintenance of your cells. (Why these patients deal with a lot of depression and no, SSRIs don't always work with them.)

> ➤ You'll also make glutathione through this proper methylation pathway. For example, if you create more glutathione it means you will have a better chance in eliminating toxins and heavy metals, which can reduce your risk for cancer, other health issues, and put less stress on your adrenals.

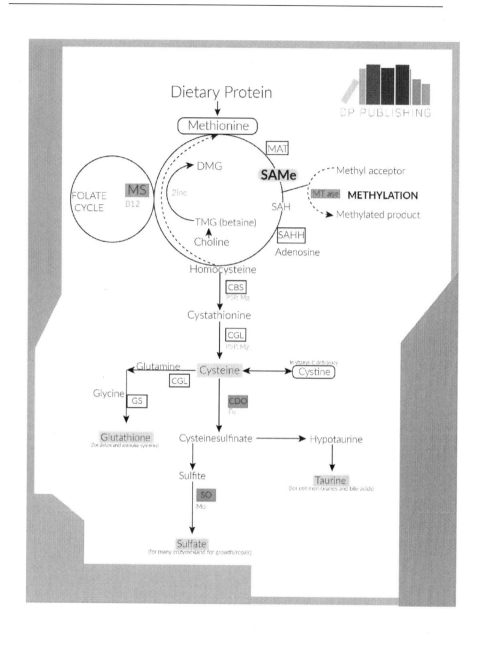

And from the National Library of Medicine we learn[4]:

> *"The official name of this gene is "methylenetetrahydrofolate reductase (NAD(P)H)."*

MTHFR is the gene's official symbol.

SAMe, which we'll discuss later, is made of methionine. And with the MTHFR enzyme deficiency (which is what we're talking about here) you may not be able to make methionine or SAMe, so you may be suffering from a SAMe deficiency also. But there's a way to cut through what used to be a lot of testing – and I'll show you how.

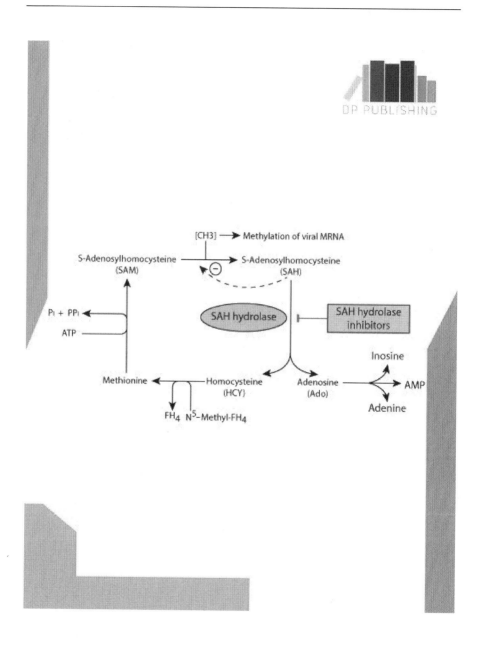

Read on.

3

WHAT A DEFECTIVE (MUTATED) MTHFR GENE DOES TO YOU

(Some of this was borrowed from this EXCELLENT website – please go there - *http://www.stopthethyroidmadness.com/mthfr/*)

WHAT DOES A defective MTHFR gene structure do to you?[5]

➢ It causes a reduction in the production of the critical MTHFR enzyme, causing methylation to occur at only 40% of a healthy body's capacity, or even as much as 70% of its capacity (still bad though). It can mean you could have been diagnosed with heavy metal toxicity – you won't break down toxins or heavy metals fast enough – i.e. you could find yourself with high iron, or high copper, or high lead, or high mercury....etc. High copper can also cause low ferritin, even though your iron levels look great (take natural Vitamin C to lower copper levels in this case – but your Spectracell® Metabolic Panel will have probably have shown you have a Vitamin C deficiency at this point)!

- The defective enzyme doesn't break down folate vitamins properly (of which folic acid is the precursor to), which can cause high homocysteine levels (hyperhomocysteinuria), which causes vascular inflammation which in turn can increase your risk of coronary heart disease (arteriosclerotic vascular disease or venous thrombosis), and related heart and high BP conditions, as well as increasing your risk for dementia. (This vascular inflammation can explain why someone young has high blood pressure of unknown cause—in turn when treated, their BP should drop to normal).

- Homocysteine is then inadequately converted to glutathione, which is your body's chief antioxidant and detoxifier. You are then more susceptible to fatigue, stress and toxin buildup (see the chapter on glutathione for more info).

- Homocysteine is poorly converted to methionine, and less methionine can raise your risk of arteriosclerosis, fatty liver degenerative disease, anemia, increased inflammation, increased free radical damage... and produce less SAMe.

- Less SAMe can increase depression (another reason why these patients have high levels of depression – this is most appropriately treated with vitamins, not anti-depressants).

- You can become toxic with high folate or high B12 levels, i.e. your body will have problems converting inactive forms of folate and B12 to the active forms. So the inactive folate or B12 will simply build up in your serum, also inhibiting the active forms. Most serum folate tests are actually measuring folic acid, which needed to be converted to methylfolate to be used metabolically.

MORE THAN ONE TRANSCRIPTION ERROR OF THE MTHFR GENE

Genes are passed down by your mother and your father. Most literature states there are a good 40-50 different mutations of this important gene which could be passed down by one, or both of your parents. But only three are particularly problematic: transcription errors (it's technically *not a mutation* but a copying or transcription error) on the points at C677T and A1298C, and to a lesser degree COMT. The 677 and 1298 numbers refer to their location on the first gene. You will also sometimes just see them written as just 677 and 1298.

There are multiple potential combinations of MTHFR:

- ➤ **Homozygous**: means you have both copies of either the 677 error, or the 1298 error, since you're getting one from each parent.

- ➤ **Heterozygous**: means you have one copy of either the 677 error, or the 1298 error, plus a normal one from the other parent. For example - C677T error alone can cause a decrease of 40% in your methylation capabilities.

- ➤ **Compound Heterozygous**: means you have one copy of the 677 error from one parent and one copy of the 1298 error from the other parent.

- ➤ **Triple homozygous errors** (more rare): an example would be one C677T, one A1298C, and a P39P or R594Q,.

Here are the possible combinations:

- Normal/Normal for both 677 and 1298
- Heterozygous 1298 / Normal 677 (one parent passed down a single 1298 error)—No symptoms
- Homozygous 1298 / Normal 677 (both parents passed down the 1298 mutation) - severe symptoms – the worst?
- Heterozygous 677 / Normal 1298 (one parent passed down a single 677 mutation) – mild symptoms.
- Homozygous 677 / Normal 1298 (both parents passed down the 677 mutation) – severe symptoms.
- Heterozygous 677 / Homozygous 1298 (one parent passed down the 677 mutation; both passed down the 1298) – bad mental symptoms etc.
- Homozygous 677 / Heterozygous 1298 (both parents passed down the 677 mutation; one passed down the 1298) – severe symptoms.
- Heterozygous 677 / Heterozygous 1298 (Compound Heterozygous: one parent passed down the 677; one passed down the 1298) – moderate symptoms.
- Homozygous 677 / Homozygous 1298 (Compound Homozygous, both parents passed down, meaning you have two 677, two 1298) – the worst of the worst symptoms. It's hard to treat.

4

TWO TAKES ON LIVING WITH MTHFR

46 YEAR OLD CAUCASIAN HISPANIC MIX FEMALE STORY (IN IIER OWN WORDS)

"My first pregnancy was during my 20th year of life. I had been married nearly two years and this was a much anticipated pregnancy. As the beginning weeks came on, I found myself violently ill with hypergravaderium...

Completely unable to keep food and water down, let alone the prenatal vitamins. Of course I over-worried about birth defects etc due to malnutrition, and lack of prenatal vitamins. My physician ordered IV drips during all my pregnancies, which included a vitamin B regime and phenergan. It was such an amazing boost to get those methylated vitamin Bs via the IV and I was instantly revived, ready to go physically, mentally and emotionally. From this point on I was able to keep meals down, so I made great effort to choose whole foods to give my babies a fighting chance without being able to tolerate prenatals.

I believe my fibromyalgia is also related to years of not getting adequate b's in my vitamin supplementation, even with the heroic efforts I have made in my actual diet. Identifying that I do, yes in fact, have MTHFR (Compound Hetrozygous or one of each error – plus I'm an "over-methylator so I have to be careful with SAMe which makes me feel horrible), treating it daily with proper vitamin supplements (using just two Homocystex™ Plus a day – I cannot go higher) and a whole food diet, my daily life has increased dramatically – energy, activity and productivity wise. It is a mental relief as well after being told for years by western physicians (which Dr. Purser admits he is with "a touch of naturopath") that they couldn't see what was wrong with me, therefore unable to do anything for me other than write a prescription for depression, or suggest an amphetamine. and one for narcotics for aches and pains. I always said "no thank you."

24 YEAR OLD CAUCASIAN MALE STORY IN HIS OWN WORDS

LIVING WITH MTHFR

"I am a 24-year-old male that has the homozygous C677T MTHFR gene transcription error. I was only recently diagnosed with this mutation. Several years ago I learned that I had extremely low testosterone serum levels, and along with this came all the symptoms of low testosterone. For years I dealt with "depression," never being able to fully focus on any subjects in school. My mind was cloudy most of the day and I was tired all the time. The only time I felt happy was when I went to Disneyland, but even there I would get tired by noon and have to rest. Again, I was a teenager and should have had plenty of energy. I never understood just how messed up I was. I always had the thought that you just have to suffer through it and make the best of it. Sure you can do that, but why, when you can feel good?

I never had deep desires to pursue anything. I also always struggled with my weight. I never felt good enough to actively pursue a healthy lifestyle. I didn't have energy to work out other than minimal physical activity in Marching Band.

With low testosterone I also had bad vitamin levels. I always had low Vitamin B and tried taking supplements but either got sick from it and my levels would not get any better. It wasn't until just a couple months ago that I went to Dr. Purser and he informed me of MTHFR and made the connection to my low testosterone. With my type of mutation, I could not process Vitamin B on a cellular level, leading to extremely low levels of testosterone and only 30% MTHFR enzyme production efficiency.

I now am taking the product Homocysteine Supreme™ everyday along with other vitamin supplements and I am feeling great. I recently had my testosterone levels checked again, and they were higher than they have been in a very long time. My mind is clear and as I am in college, I am able to focus in my classes and study well for exams. I also have desire to exercise much more frequently that I ever had. My life has changed, and I only hope it continues to improve, now knowing the root cause of my health issues."

THE WOMAN CONTINUES...

Her Spectracell™ Comprehensive Micronutrient Panel results had returned and it was no surprise – she had several interesting intracellular deficiencies – B12, B6, Zinc, pantothenate, CoQ10, glutathione, and she was borderline deficient for magnesium and copper. These deficiencies were very problematic and would cause anyone to be extremely fatigued, but more importantly they indicated something deeper.

I had my staff call her in.

A week later she showed up. The "reveal" was always fun – this was undoubtedly a life-long problem that those who were suffering from did not even consider or know enough to ask questions regarding it. So this meeting was life altering. The Human Genome Project had only been completed in 2003, and it was from which this information really stemmed. It was all so futuristic. Hard for people to get their heads around.

This would be her case today. She was sick.

She sat down across from me – she still looked sad. And beat up.

Haggard would have been a word I would have used when I was younger, but now to my older more experienced eyes, she just looked old and tired before her time.

"Your labs came back." I slid her a copy. She looked at it.

I continued. "It's about what I thought, but it's not good."

She looked up and held the results out, "Can you explain this to me?"

"Those are some pretty serious intracellular vitamin deficiencies. Any normal person would be exhausted if they had just one of those and you have several. And they've been going on for a long time. You should be dragging."

"Then this is good? I mean I though I ate pretty good – all natural. But if I take care of these I'll get a LOT better?"

I shuffled through her labs and then looked at her. "Amazingly so, but it's not that easy."

She looked me in the eyes – a question on her face. "So how long do you think these have been going on?"

"In your life – forever."

"You mean I was born with these?"

"I think so."

"How?"

"I'm not a 100% sure but I strongly suspect you have a genetic condition called MTHFR – really MTHFR Enzyme Deficiency Disease – it's a disorder causing you to not be able to methylate properly – a function of your body that adds energy. This is why you're tired all the time. I think you've had these deficiencies since you were a baby. You're lucky you're alive still and not handicapped."

She digested what I just said. The air the room was thick. I could almost see her mind work through it.

"So this is why I was tired all throughout high school and junior high? Why I always need naps?"

I nodded.

"My dad just thought I was lazy. I'd catch hell."

"Sorry but your dad probably had to give you half this problem."

She nodded. "How do we know for sure? And how do you treat this? Can you?"

"We need to test your genetics. Spectracell® can run that too. Just one little tube of blood. Takes a couple of weeks – we send it to Texas. Different genetic patterns need to be treated slightly differently – some more differently. Plus I am not 100% sure you have this – just an educated guess."

"What else could it be?"

"Just bad vitamin deficiencies. But this pattern leads me, like footprints in the sand, to conclude that you have this disorder – seen this dozens of time. So, I'm not wrong."

She nodded. Still digesting. "What next?"

"We draw your blood for the genetic testing. I'll also start you on some vitamins for this condition – but they're not the kind you can buy at just any grocery store."

She raised an eyebrow.

"These vitamins have been "manipulated" to work around the enzyme deficiencies you might or do have. Some really smart people made them."

"Like you? Don't you design stuff?"

"Not like these," I said. "These were super smart people."

She nodded. Smiled.

"Also, they'll look like someone read the future and designed them almost exactly for your Spectracell® results – like they knew in advance."

"Humphhh..."

"Yeah, cool, eh?"

I handed her a bottle of Powerful Mind™ and said, "Start on this – one a day for a week then two. We always start low and go slow."

"Why?"

"Picture yourself as a methyl well that's only half full. When your full of methyl groups your energy level is perfect – it will be amazing. If we ever overfill it you will crash."

"So what happens if I overmethylate?"

"Crazy symptoms. High anxiety or panic sets in, hyperactivity, rapid speech, low libido, nervous legs, pacing, dry eyes and mouth, low motivation, depression, self mutilation, sleep problems, tinnitus, facial hair, food/chemical sensitivities, and stuff like that."

She looked horrified.

"So we don't want that."

"No we don't. But how quickly will I improve?"

"Not quickly if we do it right, however if we stay steady it will improve slowly but surely. You can search for all this stuff and various patient blogs online."

It all sank in.

"Take one of those Powerful Mind™ capsules a day to begin with and every week add another one – call me immediately if any problems." I slid her my card it had all my contact info on it.

"Want to draw your labs?"

"Okay, well let's do this."

I followed her to the lab draw room.

5

POTENTIAL DISEASES OR CONDTIONS CAUSED BY MTHFR MUTATIONS[6]

This is a fairly comprehensive list of diseases and conditions caused by or associated with MTHFR gene mutations (again most are borrowed from MTHFR.net, though over the years I've added a few here and there):

1. Autism (95-98%+ have two snps – the actual MTHFR disease)
2. DVT (deep venous thrombosis or leg clots)
3. Down's Syndrome
4. Miscarriages

5. Pernicious Anemia

6. Gluten Intolerance

7. Neural Tube Defects

8. Pulmonary Embolisms

9. Depression in Post-Menopausal Women

10. Schizophrenia

11. Fibromyalgia

12. Chronic Fatigue Syndrome

13. Exhaustion

14. Chemical Sensitivity

15. Parkinson's Disease

16. Irritable Bowel Syndrome

17. Pre-eclampsia

18. Stroke

19. Spina Bifida

20. Esophageal Squamous Cell Carcinoma

21. Acute Lymphoblastic Leukemia

22. Vascular Dementia

23. Bipolar Disorder

24. Colorectal Adenoma

25. Idiopathic Male Infertility

26. Blood Clots

27. Rectal Cancer

28. Meningioma

29. Glioma

30. Congenital Heart Defects

31. Infant Depression Via Epigenetic Processes Caused By Maternal Depression

32. Deficits in Childhood Cognitive Development
33. Gastric Cancer
34. Migraines with Aura
35. Low HDL
36. High Homocysteine
37. Post-Menopausal Breast Cancer
38. Atherosclerosis
39. Oral Clefts
40. Type 1 Diabetes
41. Epilepsy
42. Primary Closed Angle Glaucoma
43. Alzheimer's Disease
44. Tetralogy of Fallot
45. Decreased Telomere Length
46. Potential Drug Toxicities: Methotrexate, Anti-Epileptics
47. Cervical Dysplasia
48. Increased Bone Fracture Risk in Post-Menopausal Women
49. Multiple Sclerosis
50. Essential Hypertension
51. Differentiated Thyroid Carcinoma
52. Prostate Cancer
53. Premature Death
54. Placental Abruption
55. Myocardial Infarction (Heart Attack)
56. Methotrexate Toxicity
57. Nitrous Oxide Toxicity
58. Heart Murmurs

59. Tight Anal Sphincters
60. Tongue Tie
61. Midline Defects (many are listed above)
62. Behcet's Disease
63. Ischemic Stroke in Children
64. Unexplained Neurologic Disease
65. Asthma
66. Shortness of Breath
67. Bladder Cancer
68. Anencephaly
69. Hypotestosteronism
70. Heavy Metal Toxicity

6

THINGS TO AVOID WHEN YOU HAVE MTHFR

1. Folic Acid – it's synthetic and is toxic to MTHFR patients. It's the first thing I tell my patients to avoid and to learn to read the labels as they search for it.

2. Cyanocobalamin – it's made with cyanide and is cheap, and also tends to be toxic to MTHFR patients. Please, use a natural form of methylcobalamin.

3. Birth control pills (BCPs) and methotrexate (for arthritis) block folate uptake in the gut. Women who take BCPs will feel like they've entered hell and will just be miserable, and won't know why.

4. Avoid taking proton pump inhibitors (PPIs) such as Prilosec™ or Prevacid™ or most antacids, which tend to block essential Vitamin B12 absorption in the gut.[7]

5. If your homocysteine level is elevated, limit your intake of methionine-rich foods (high methionine foods include nuts, beef, lamb, cheese, turkey, pork, fish, shellfish, soy, eggs, dairy, and beans).[8] The recommended daily intake for

methionine is 10.4mg per kilogram of body weight, or 4.5mg per pound.

6. Avoid eating processed foods, many of which have added synthetic folic acid (a substance toxic to MTHFR enzyme deficient patients). Instead, try to eat whole foods with no added chemicals or preservatives (see the diet book we wrote for these patients MTHFR WHOLE FOOD COOKBOOK & MEAL PLANS 2016).

7. Get your daily intake of leafy greens, like spinach, kale, swiss chard, or arugula, (add broccoli too) which are loaded with natural folate (in the form of folic acid) which is a form that your body can more easily process.

8. Because you probably can't make adequate amounts of glutathione (which is the substance our body uses to remove heavy metals) remove any mercury amalgams with a trained biologic or naturopathic dentist. Avoiding heavy metal or other toxic exposure is important.

9. Make sure you supplement with essential nutrients, like B12 (methylcobalamin), natural folate (methylfolate, NatureFolate©, or even folic acid or Quatrefolic©), TMG, N-acetylcysteine, riboflavin, curcumin, fish oil, Vitamin C (natural form of it), D (cholecalcifereol or D3 in a liquid-gel – not the dry form), E (mixed alpha-tocopherols), and probiotics. If you are double homozygous for MTHFR mutations (especially C677T), you should proceed very cautiously with methyl-B12 and methyl-folate supplementation as some people do not tolerate high doses. Introduce nutrients one by one, watching for any adverse reactions. Use extreme caution when supplementing with niacin, which can dampen methylation.

10. Avoid eating a lot of copper or foods that contain copper and conversely eat more zinc containing foods.[9]

11. Avoid taking aspirin or enalaprin (i.e. Lovenox™ – I'm not sure why to avoid this but have been told to use

nattokinase instead to thin blood (more natural) – I cannot find a reference in the literature but have been told this at more than one meeting – maybe it's just an old doctor's tale?

12. Birth Control Pills or Depo-Provera™. Why? Because MTHFR patien's or sufferers already have an increased risk of clotting and thrombophilia, and these medicines can shove them over the threshold.[10]

13. Folic acid. What? Yes – this is synthetic. 5-Methyl-Tetrahydrofolate or 5-MTF-Quatrafolic Acid or folinic acid are all okay, too - just never folic acid. Be careful even ingesting it in multi-vitamins or processed foods.

14. PRENATAL VITAMINS. If you're a pregnant woman and prenatal vitamins make you ill, it may be because of the high load of folic acid but it could also be a lack of the MTHFR enzyme.

7

PROPER MTHFR THERAPIES

TAKING B VITAMINS in the face of an MTHFR gene mutation can sometimes lead to nausea and high homocysteine levels (hyperhomocysteinemia) – both big problems (but also diagnostic clues for the astute patient and/or physician).

You need to think of this genetic illness as a disease where you have a "methylation well" that has never been full before. Never in your whole life has it been full. This is the well from which you draw methyl groups to make energy (in the citric acid cycle) or glutathione and other vitamins to detox and make hormones. The goal in therapy is to fill this well up with methyl groups – at 100% full your energy level is optimal – this is what a properly treated MTHFR deficient patient feels and they are truly amazed at how good they feel (that's what this book is about). These MTHFR deficient patients are also usually (not always) off of anti-depressants and even BP meds and hormones such as testosterone.

So what happens IF you ever overfill this methylation well? They will enter a world of hurt and depression and other odd symptoms. Do NOT overfill the Methylation well. It is a hard and tricky pathway on which to travel and the patient (you) needs to know this as you begin. And the pathway is full of all kinds of options and erroneous choices – it can be hard to maneuver.

To properly treat (or to back into the diagnosis properly) you must obtain both a SpectraCell® Comprehensive Micronutrient Analysis (it's an intracellular vitamin and mineral test) and proper gene testing (which can also be done through SpectraCell®). As pricey as this is, this test allows you leap past a LOT of enzyme testing, causing you to hopefully see the exact intracellular vitamin deficiencies possibly caused by the genetic defects or mutations (I say possibly because the deficiency could just be by chance – MTHFR defects do not always cause an intracellular vitamin deficiency), and then also the genetic mutation (A1298C versus C677T or both) – either of which or a combination of which potentially changes the treatment options.

METHIONINE OR MEAT RESTRICTED DIETS

Methionine restriction is recommended for risk variant carriers to reduce homocysteine accumulation and limit the effects of reduced MTHFR activity. Since dietary methionine is mostly found in animal proteins, and folate is mainly found in vegetables, methionine restriction calls for vegetarian-oriented diets. In vegetarian diet regimens, a vitamin B12 (as methylcoblamin supplement is strongly recommended since it is primarily found in animal products.[11]

PROPER "MANIPULATED" VITAMINS

Once these determinations are made, the patient can be given certain molecularly "manipulated" vitamins that can be absorbed around the mutation or defect. The patient will notice improvement within a month or so.

I look for a combination vitamin that contains:

Vitamin B6 (pyridoxine and P5P blend)

Folate

5-MTHF (Methyltetrahyrdofolate)

5-FTHF (folinic acid)

Pantothenic acid

Vitamin B12 (as methylcobalamin)

Zinc chelate

Amino Acids (that contains at least Serine, Glutamine, NACA, Tyrosine, and Glycine as TrimethylGlycine or TMG)

If nausea occurs, I'd also add 25 mg of Niacin (or more).

You should be able to find these from your doctor or online.

8

METHYLATION SUPPPORT

MY FAVORITE PRODUCT FOR MTHFR

Is there a perfect vitamin for MTHFR Enzyme Deficiency?

Clearly, no.

This is a complex problem affected by many other genetic issues that are underneath the MTHFR transcription errors – as I've said before - we humans now probably contain hundreds of mutations and transcription errors – MTHFR is just the most obvious. So trying to design a "multi-vitamin" or many faceted product that fits all is very difficult, if not impossible.

I'd design it to fill as many methylation issues or to fill as many of the usual vitamin and mineral holes as MTHFR deficiency typically causes.

When you look at the lab results, where I show Spectracell™ Comprehensive Micronutrient Panel results later, you'll see what I mean.

Again, here is my MUST CONTAIN list:

Vitamin B6 (pyridoxine and P5P blend)

Folate

5-MTHF (Methyltetrahyrdofolate)

5-FTHF (folinic acid)

Pantothenic acid

Vitamin B12 (as methylcobalamin)

Zinc chelate

Amino Acids (that contains at least Serine, Glutamine, NACA, Tyrosine, and Glycine as TrimethylGlycine or TMG)

BUT, all this said, this has to be a vitamin that comes in a small dose so it can be adjusted up slowly. I'd limit the folate to 1000 mcg a capsule, the 5-MTHF (methyltetrahydrafolate) to 1000 mcg, and the methylcobalamin to 500 mcg. Some patients may be able to take 1/day and some will want to work up to taking 8/day.

A LITTLE ABOUT HOMOCYSTEINE

Let's call the above conglomeration of vitamins and nutrients "methylation support" nutrients (vitamin B6 and B12), including proprietary NatureFolate™ blend of active isomer naturally-occurring folates, known to assist in the metabolism of homocysteine in the face of MTHFR genetic enzyme errors. That blend would help assist in allowing a more healthy homocysteine pathway (often for the first time in a MTHFR patient's life), allowing for the normal production of all the steps in the pathway.

Let's look at the pathway again:

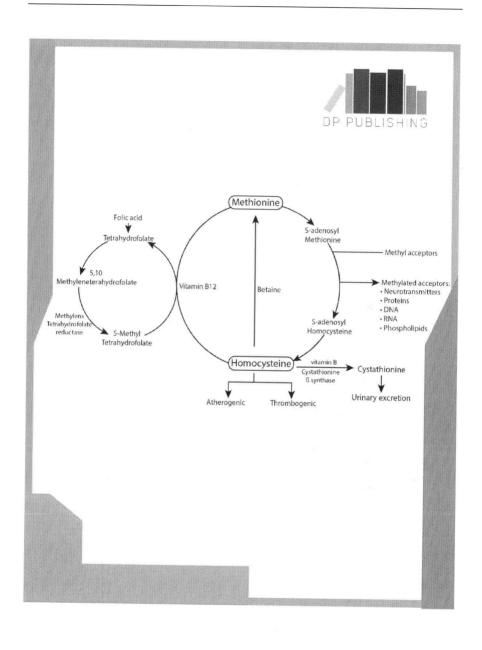

These amino acids should include the sulfur-containing amino acids taurine and cysteine.

An optimally functioning homocysteine pathway provides methyl and sulfur groups for a number of biochemical reactions such as detoxification (glutathione production), immune function, ideal joint and cartilage structure, and brain and cardiovascular health.

What is Homocysteine?

Homocysteine is a sulfur-containing amino acid produced in the body during the metabolism of the essential amino acid methionine, which involves a series of conversions that require enzymes (again see the above diagram), many of which can be affected by the enzyme deficiencies incurred by MTHFR genetic errors. Homocysteine is a natural substance which we need and should not be feared, but appreciated and controlled. Homocysteine functions at a metabolic crossroad and who's errors in manufacturing or utilization can affect the methyl and sulfur group metabolism of key enzymes, hormones, and vital nutrients – this is one of the reasons why I see such low testosterone levels (and other hormones) in these MTHFR patients. Many important nutrients, especially B vitamins, are needed for these enzymes, but again are unable to be used properly in an intracellular manner due to the MTHFR.

The Problem with too much Homocysteine[12]

The circulation of excess homocysteine causes significant inflammation damaging the lining of arterial walls so they become narrow and inelastic, and blood pressure increases[13]. Research suggests that a raised homocysteine level is an independent risk factor for hardening of the arteries, coronary heart disease, stroke, peripheral vascular disease, and other conditions associated with abnormal blood clotting.

Elevated homocysteine is also linked with a number of other serious medical conditions including osteoporosis, Alzheimer's disease, multiple sclerosis, rheumatoid arthritis, spontaneous abortion, placental abruption, renal failure, and type II diabetes. When homocysteine is elevated it reduces nitric oxide (NO) production via increasing levels of asymmetric dimethyl-arginine (ADMA)[14], which can increase the risk of hypertension and erectile dysfunction.

You need a blend (i.e. "methylation support") that will assist in the appropriate metabolism of homocysteine, thus preventing toxic levels of homocysteine from accumulating. This makes it possible for a functioning methylation pathway to provide necessary methyl and sulfur groups for a all of those biochemical reactions pictured in the above diagram, especially those needed for detoxification, joint and cartilage repair, and brain health.[15]

How and how often should we test homocysteine levels and other vitamin levels?

Individuals with a personal or family history of coronary heart disease, or other CHD risk factors, or who have the MTHFR (methyltetrahydrofolate reductase) genetic error should have homocysteine testing at least twice per year.

Testing for key vitamin deficiencies should be done on an intracellular level at least once a year once in treatment, and levels of folic acid, B6 and B12 are very easy via bloodspot and/or urine collection. The Spectracell® is the only option for this type of testing and cuts many corners that other physicians are suggesting, and saves a lot of money.

Elevations of any of these markers on the comprehensive metabolic profile (CMP) test may increase risk of homocysteinemia.[16]   Individuals with hypothyroidism (and many patients with MTHFR have hypothyroidism) are at greater risk of hyperhomocysteinemia, because hypothyroidism decreases hepatic levels of enzymes involved in the remethylation pathway of homocysteine.[17]

How do we know that correcting these deficiencies will help longevity?

A meta-analysis of 12 randomized controlled trials suggested that supplementation with 0.5-5.7 mg folic acid per day could reduce elevated homocysteine levels by 25%, while adding 0.02-1 mg per day vitamin B12 produced a further 7% reduction.[18] In a study of 350 elderly people aged 65-75 years, folic acid supplements of 400-600mcg per day were needed to produce significant lowering of homocysteine levels compared to placebo.

Due to reduced absorption in the elderly, it was estimated that a total intake of 926mcg per day was needed to avoid folate deficiency and lower cardiovascular risk.

The addition of vitamin B12 is doubly important here, as folate can mask early signs of vitamin B12 deficiency which might lead to subacute combined degeneration of the spinal cord.[19]

Have researchers yet done large-scale trials to assess whether interventions to lower homocysteine levels will reduce cardiovascular morbidity and mortality?

One recent analysis suggested that supplementation of B vitamins did not reduce risk of cardiovascular events. This conclusion should not be considered valid because the subjects had previous cardiovascular events, and the doses were not high enough for positive results considering the age of the subjects, as just discussed.

There is adequate evidence that controlling homocysteine, and adequately supplementing folic acid and B12 will improve overall health, reduce cardiovascular risk and increase longevity.

Even older women need higher doses of B vitamins. After menopause, some women are less able to process homocysteine, which may explain the higher risk of coronary heart disease in this group.

Hormone replacement therapies, as well as oral contraceptives, deplete B vitamins. A survey in the US suggested that only 40-50% of people obtained enough folic acid from their diet to process homocysteine normally.

Do individuals with the faulty MTHFR genotype need to take 5,10 methyltetrahydrofolate, which is more expensive than folic acid?

No. Research shows that supplementation of folic acid gets better homocysteine lowering results than supplementing 5,10 MTHF in individuals with this faulty genotype and in the other genotypes as well.[20] Methylenetetrahydrofolate reductase enzyme (MTHFR) catalyzes the synthesis of 5-methyltetrahydrofolate (5-MTHF), the methyl donor for the formation of methionine from homocysteine. Research does not support the belief that having this gene polymorphism means these individuals have poor folic acid metabolism.

One particular study looked at the ability of homozygotes for the MTHFR C677T (this CT genotype mutates to TT) to convert 5-formyltetrahydrofolic acid (folinic acid) to 5-MTHF, a process that requires the action of the MTHFR enzyme. These researchers concluded that the conversion of oral folinic acid to 5-MTHF is not impaired in persons with the mutated T/T MTHFR genotype.[21]

A quote from Kelly in the Alternative Medicine Review says:

> "Administration of folinic acid bypasses the deconjugation and reduction steps required for folic acid. Folinic acid also appears to be a more metabolically active form of folate, capable of boosting levels of the coenzyme forms of the vitamin in circumstances where folic acid has little to no effect. Therapeutically, folic acid can reduce homocysteine levels and the occurrence of neural tube defects, might play a role in preventing cervical dysplasia and protecting against neoplasia in ulcerative colitis, appears to be a rational aspect of a nutritional protocol to treat vitiligo, and can increase the resistance of the gingiva to local irritants, leading to a reduction in inflammation. Reports also indicate that neuropsychiatric diseases secondary to folate deficiency might include dementia, schizophrenia-like syndromes, insomnia, irritability, forgetfulness, endogenous depression, organic psychosis, peripheral neuropathy, myelopathy, and restless legs syndrome."[22]

Another study involving hemodialysis (HD) individuals showed folinic acid supplementation significantly reduced hyperhomocysteinaemia, MDA (Malondialdehyde) levels, and oxidized LDL.

Quoted here is the author's conclusion: Treatment with folinic acid lowers plasma homocysteine levels and, like vitamin E, affords antioxidant protection, which prevents lipid peroxidation. This lowering of lipid peroxidation may reduce the risk of atherosclerosis and prevent or delay cardiovascular complications in HD individuals.[23] So, in a nutshell, folinic acid, supplied in Homocysteine Supreme, is an active form of a group of vitamins known as folates. Folinic acid is one of the forms of folate (bound to calcium) found naturally in foods. Folate deficiency is believed to be the most common vitamin deficiency in the world due to food processing, food selection, and intestinal disorders. In the body folinic acid may be converted into any of the other active forms of folate.

Why so much emphasis on converting homocysteine back to methionine?

Many doctors don't realize that the most common block in the homocysteine pathway is the conversion of cystathionine to cysteine which requires B6 to activate the cystathionine beta-synthase enzyme, making B6 an important ingredient in the "methylation support". B6 is also required in the step that converts homocysteine into cystathionine.[24] Serine is needed in this step as well. Remember this part of the pathway synthesizes cysteine is needed for glutathione synthesis and taurine which has multiple functions including preventing catabolism due to chronic stress and aiding insulin function, both being important for our metabolic syndrome individuals.

This "methylation support" formula (by supplying folates and methylcobalamin B12) does aid the process for homocysteine to be converted back to methionine in case the body is in need of converting methionine into SAMe (S-adenosylmethionine) which is known to improve depression, synthesize neurotransmitters and support joint comfort, function and mobility in the spine, hips and knees. It is important to the joints because of its critical role in cartilage production.

If SAMe is supplemented in the absence of adequate B12, homocysteine levels may increase.

Besides faulty enzymes and genes are there chemicals that cause faulty methionine conversion?

Yes, heavy metals. Mercury and lead are known to bind to these sulfur amino acids and interfere with the pathway. Mercury depletes B12 and may interfere also by causing a deficiency of this key methylator. The methylcobalamin form of B12 is responsible for remethylating folic acid so it can convert homocysteine back to methionine. However, too much emphasis on converting the pathway backwards does not allow the body to synthesize more cysteine if needed.

Mercury toxicity creates a greater need for cysteine and glutathione – more on this later but you need an absorbable, reduced, stable glutathione (called GSH) for this problem. Chronic mercury inhalation from mercury fillings, with its great affinity to bind to sulfur amino acids, methionine and cysteine, can decrease the availability of these amino acids and affect the metabolism of both vitamin B12 and folic acid, making higher supplemental doses crucial.

Cysteine is needed to synthesize glutathione, the most important antioxidant in the human body. High amounts of glutathione are used up to protect the body from heavy metals such as mercury. Glutathione helps the liver to detoxify chemicals. This antioxidant prevents apoptosis, dying of our cells due to excessive oxidative stress caused by heavy metals and chemicals, especially a problem in people who do not consume enough fruits and vegetables, which contain antioxidants.[25]

9

WHAT IS TMG?[26]

TRIMETHYLGLYCINE OR TMG is a vitamin-like substance. It functions as an anti-oxidant, anti-inflammatory, energy booster, methyl donor and more. It is also commonly deficient in MTHFR sufferers.

TMG is also called betaine because it was first isolated from sugar beets. It is not the same as betaine hydrochloride, however. It should be added to most all-nutritional balancing programs, usually in doses of 1000-3000 mg daily. Some people need even more, especially when moving through healing reactions. Most people seem to need it and benefit greatly from it. It does not seem to interfere with the rest of a nutritional balancing program, which is very unusual.

Many people do not make enough TMG today. The reason appears to be the presence of certain toxic metals. In addition, stress, infections, inflammation, and other disease conditions may use up what the body makes, so more is needed.

Sources Of TMG

1. Plenty of TMG is made in a healthy body.
2. Some can also be obtained from the diet.
3. One can take it as a food supplement that is available in many health food stores.

Dietary sources of TMG. The main foods high in TMG are broccoli, beets and other vegetables. These foods are naturally high in TMG and in folate, which are both methyl donors. The problem is that most people do not eat nearly enough of these foods to get a sufficient amount of TMG from their diet. Also, even if one eats plenty of these vegetables, it is not nearly enough. So I suggest supplementing it as well.

Supplements. Supplementary TMG appears to be very helpful due to 1) low production inside the body, 2) a greater need for TMG today, and 3) inadequate dietary intake of TMG. See below for dosages, and cautions with supplementary TMG.

The Basic Structure Of TMG

TMG consists of three methyl groups (CH3) joined to one molecule of the amino acid glycine. This is a very important type of structure because, when eaten in food or taken orally as a supplement, TMG easily lets go of two or even three of its methyl groups.

Letting go of one methyl group leaves a substance called dimethylglycine or DMG. Letting go of three methyl groups frees up a molecule of the amino acid glycine.

Functions Of TMG

TMG is MAJORLY useful for the body as a methyl donor. In addition, it has other uses when broken down into DMG and glycine, or transformed into SAMe or other compounds such as methionine. Let us discuss a few of these.

A powerful and safe methyl donor. TMG easily donates three methyl groups to the body. Methyl groups (CH3) are required in millions of biochemical reactions in human and animal bodies. Here are just a few of the best studied examples:

1. Lowering homocysteine

Homocysteine is an amino acid that, in excess, is irritating to the arteries and is strongly associated with inflammation and hardening of the arteries. In fact, the level of homocysteine correlates more closely with heart disease than the level of cholesterol.

Doctors are beginning to realize this important link. High homocysteine occurs when there is not enough TMG or folic acid to donate enough methyl groups. There can be other causes, but this is the major cause. As explained earlier, a deeper cause for this is the presence of mercury and copper toxicity, which are almost universal. However, the problem can be solved with a diet high in TMG and folate, or a TMG or folate supplement. One does not need both in most cases.

High homocysteine, however, causes many other problems. It causes a deficiency of methionine, and this, in turn, can cause a deficiency of SAMe, causing depression in some people. Methionine is also needed for other biochemical reactions involving protein synthesis, another critical body function. In fact, reducing excessive homocysteine helps with conditions ranging from osteoporosis and birth defects to cancer and aging. It also helps with antioxidant protection, as well.

2. Helping with liver detoxification

Methyl groups are absolutely essential for the Phase 2, Cytochrome P450 liver detoxification pathway. Within this critical biochemical sequence of events, fat-soluble or otherwise poorly soluble toxins that are difficult for the liver to remove are joined to a methyl group, and this helps prepare them for removal from the body. This is an amazing and vital chemical detoxification ability. In MOST people, it does not work well due living in a very toxic world.

Specifically, the methylation reaction enables toxins to become much more soluble in water. This allows the body to remove the toxins much better, and it often neutralizes some of their toxic properties as well. These toxins include all of the toxic metals in many forms and compounds, as well as hundreds of toxic chemicals. Much more could be written about this amazing system and how critical it is today for our health. This is one of the main benefits of TMG supplementation, I believe.

3. Alleviating depression

TMG increases the body's natural production of SAMe or S-adenosyl methionine. This chemical can help reduce depression, in some cases. SAMe is an expensive supplement, and a more yin supplement, which is not good. It appears to be far better to just take TMG.

4. Reducing the chances of diabetes

Methyl groups are involved in insulin release and insulin activity. When the body does not have enough active methyl groups, diabetes is much more likely to arise.

5. Avoiding genetic problems

Methyl groups are needed for protein synthesis, also called biosynthesis. This is the copying of our genetic code from the DNA to RNA, and then from there the synthesis or formation of every chemical in our bodies. The copying of the DNA is also called genetic transcription.

Without enough TMG, biosynthesis can slow down, telomeres can shorten, and genetic errors, also called transcription errors, multiply, and health is definitely worse.

Dosage And Cautions With TMG

For adults, TMG comes in tablets or capsules of 500, 750 and 1000 mg... I will often start with low doses of methionine first 200 -500 mg a day.

IMPORTANT NOTE: Do not take DMG or dimethylglycine. Only take trimethylglycine or TMG.

Dosage. Most adults need about 1000-3000 mg daily. However, some people need up to 4500 mg daily, at least for a while. Fortunately, if one takes too much, usually one does not feel well. Symptoms of too much TMG include some fatigue, nausea, hair loss, dizziness, spaciness, or rarely other symptoms.[27]

Another Option - Best Supplement to Take for TMG?

As I've said before, the best supplement in my armamentarium to take to supply would be a "methylation support". It's VERY good and by the time you take 2-3 each day you've received adequate amounts. But eat your broccoli and cauliflower too.

THE MTHFR WOMAN CONTINUES

I looked at her Spectracell™ Genetic testing report and blinked – it was worse than I expected - she was Homozygous for C677T.

I slid the results to her.

"This means?"

"You're homozygous for C677T – the worst combination you can get for this disorder."

So am I a mutant?"

I shook my head no. "No – not technically – you suffer from a transcription error."

She looked at me.

I continued. "But for all effects and purposes you're a mutant. Sorry."

"How does this change my treatment?"

"We can go a little faster. How did the Powerful Mind™ work?"

"It made me sleepy."

"Not unusual," I say. "But no other problems?"

She shook her head no.

"Your energy should come waaaay up with more of the right vitamins – we're filling your "methyl well." You also have Urinary Pyrrolea or Pyrrole Disease. At least your Spectracell™ vitamin panel would indicate it."

Her head came up – she looked sick.

"That just means you dump a lot of pyrroles, due to your MTHFR gene errors, into your urine. B6 and Zinc follow it – but it may take a ton of zinc to treat it. And B6."

Why is it called uhh that?"

"Urinary Pyrrolea or Pyrrole Disease? Because doctors used to think it was a stand alone disease of unknown cause, plus they found huge quantities of pyrroles in the urine of these people – I have no idea why they were looking for pyrroles in peoples' urine – and finally now we know what causes it. And how to treat it."

"Oh, just with vitamins?"

I nodded.

"Will this shorten my life expectancy?"

I nodded again. "Maybe. Experts think so. Maybe taking the right vitamins will change the numbers and risk factors, but at our age who knows what changes you can go through. We'll see."

She nodded – digesting it all.

"For now we need to check your Homocysteine level and your Whole Blood Histamine level – that last one is super important as it tells me if you're an undermethylator or overmethylator – if you need SAMe or not."

"My head's spinning."

"Sure, I'll give you my little book on this topic and get Ben Lynch's book, too, off Amazon – he's the doctor, a naturopath, who writes on MTHFR.net and is really on top of all this."

She nodded – she'd started taking notes on a little notebook.

"You've got to start educating yourself on all of this. Your responsibility, not anyone else's."

She nodded again.

"Let's go draw some more blood."

10

WHY THE 5-MTHF?

HIGH DOSE, 1000 MCG METHYLATED FOLATE, AS THE ALL NATURAL 6S ISOMER

L-5-MTHF™ is a safe and effective way to increase the body's folate levels. It is especially helpful for patients with demonstrated increased need for folate, such as those with either the A1298C or C677T MTHFR mutation.

IMPORTANT NOTE: Do not use with "UNDERMETHYLATORS" (those who have high Whole Blood Histamine Levels) as SAMe would be more beneficial. And watch for depression when you give these under-methylating patients extra folate.

This product provides 1000 mcg per capsule of folate in the bioidentical, bioactive form, 5-Methyltetrahydrofolate. L-5-

MTHF (the "L" signifying that it is the all-natural [6S] isomer) is the active circulating form of folate found in the body and one of the several forms found in food.

In nature it is found only as this [6S] isomer, which is why you should use 5-MTHF as this natural isomer rather than the mixed (or racemic) form. This innovative form of folate has demonstrated high bioavailability and solubility as well as long lasting stability. L-5-MTHF *helps to increase blood folate levels much better than folic acid.*[28]

L-5-MTHF should be used when high doses of folate are needed.

Individuals who have tested homozygous with either the A1298C or C677T MTHFR mutation, or those with elevated homocysteine levels, should be using L-5-MTHF as the preferred form of folate supplementation. This will be more effective for them than other forms of folic acid or folates.

Others who may benefit from L-5-MTHF:

> Pregnant women and women wishing to become pregnant who have familial history of depression, high homocysteine levels, or genetic defect in MTHFR. Note: Prenatal Pro™ is the Designs for Health® comprehensive multivitamin; it can be combined with L-5-MTHF if higher levels of folate are needed.

> Women with abnormal pap smears (precancerous)

> Those with very high homocysteine levels not responding to the methylation support"

> Dialysis patients

> Organic acid testing that reveals elevated FIGLU (marker sometimes used to identify folate deficiency)

> Patients with family history of dementia/vascular dementia

> ➢ Patients with depression
> ➢ Long-term alcoholism

> ➢ Long-term use of oral contraceptives, and persistent use of medications to lower folate levels, including high doses of NSAIDs such as aspirin or ibuprofen; anticonvulsants (phenytoin, phenobarbital, and primidone); trimethoprim (antibiotic), pyrimethamine (antimalarial), triamterene (blood pressure med.) and sulfasalazine (treatment for ulcerative colitis).

Do not take 5-MTHF simultaneously with the cholesterol-lowering agents cholestyramine or colestipol because they may decrease the absorption of folate.

Warning on Synthetic Folic Acid:

Read about the important differences and safety concerns to consider between Synthetic Folic vs Natural Folate™. (Designs For Health® uses Natural Folate™ in their products)

Another option, another perspective

Finding the Best Dose of Methylfolate is a Process of Trial and Error.

(This is again from Dr. Amy Neuzil a Naturopathic Doctor who's hilarious, brilliant, and very sharp – I love her work and if you need guidance on these vitamins she's a great option.)

"I wish there was just one answer – this is the right dose, but sadly it all comes down to what is the right dose for your body. First off, I never suggest taking methylfolate by itself without any other B vitamins. The B vitamins all have overlapping functions and so it's important to have decent doses of all of them. Typically though, I start clients with a B complex that has a reasonably low dose of methylfolate – like maybe 400 mcg. I really like the one from Pure Encapsulations® called B Complex Plus. It's basic, simple, and most people – even hard-core mutants – tolerate it pretty well, but I'm not married to it. Any good multi-B with a low-dose methylfolate will do or you can look for a multivitamin that has methylfolate in it like Thorne Research© Basic Nutrients®. Occasionally even this low dose creates a bad reaction – if that happens then we'll have to start with a low dose MTHF by itself and split the capsule apart but this is the option of last resort. First, let's try the low dose B complex or multivitamin and see what happens.

Keep in mind the first three days of any MTHF treatment might be difficult and there may be some adjustments. You may notice that you're a little agitated, or anxious, or depressed or just feel a little spacy or off. With any luck that should pass pretty quickly and we'll wait for things to stabilize before increasing the dose."

If the Low- MTHF B Complex or Multi Works for You

Great! We're on the right track. Even if this is the right dose for you there might be a few odd adjustment days in the beginning – that is totally normal. Just wait until everything settles down and see how you're feeling. Typically with this low dose people may notice a small spike in energy or a little boost to mood, but often it isn't enough methylfolate to start to touch the issues – that's okay because it's enough to get the ball rolling. The next step would be to add a 1 mg (1000 mcg) MTHF by itself to the B complex you're already taking. We're looking to make forward progress without rocking the boat too much. Each time you increase the dose there may be another adjustment reaction as your body gets used to things, so try to stick it out for 3 days before you make a final judgement about it.

If the Low-MTHF B Complex or Multi DOESN'T Work for You

Then we switch to plan B. Plan B is a little messier and more tedious, but it could make all the difference for how you're feeling on a day-to-day basis. Start with a 1mg MTHF – I prefer a capsule so that you can just open it and portion out the powder (instead of trying to cut or crush a tablet). In this situation start with 1/4 of the capsule – easiest is mixing it with some peanut butter, applesauce or yogurt and taking it that way. It tastes pretty gross, but hopefully you can hide it in something. Again count on about 3 days of adjustment, but we're starting with very low doses here, so hopefully that will be fine. If it's still too much then you can cut it down even further. Once you get to the dose you can tolerate, keep it there for a couple of weeks and try to slowly increase. By now your body has started to process some of the backlog of work so it might be easier to tolerate a bigger dose. Now would be a great time to try going to the B complex with MTHF or multi-vitamin with MTHF because you do still need all those other B vitamins."[29]

11

IMPORTANCE OF DETERMINING METHYLATION STATUS AND USING FOLATE VERSUS SAMe

THIS CHAPTER IS more about "life and death" – sanity versus severe depression - so it's important to understand, but if the science is too much I brought everything together at the end in a summary.

First, just because you have the symptoms, it does not mean you have the condition – you must realize that. Even if you are homozygous you still may not have any problems or symptoms or abnormalities – this is an incredibly complex interaction that has lots of manifestations. We also have lots of mutations in our bodies. Sad but true, and a critical number of them have to line up in a bad way to cause a problem. You have to have symptoms and other abnormal labs to show that a breakdown in the process has occurred – levels such as a homocysteine level, or more importantly for this chapter - a whole blood histamine level.

What's Histamine?

"Histamine is a chemical involved in your immune system, proper digestion, and your central nervous system. As a neurotransmitter, it communicates important messages from your body to your brain. It is also a component of stomach acid, which is what helps you break down food in your stomach.

Histamine causes your blood vessels to swell, or dilate, so that your white blood cells can quickly find and attack the infection or problem. The histamine buildup is what gives you a headache and leaves you feeling flushed, itchy and miserable. This is part of the body's natural immune response, but if you don't break down histamine properly, you could develop what we call histamine intolerance.

Histamine also keeps you awake (that's why anti-histamines make you sleepy) – too much histamine can drive you crazy and make you super restless. And depressed – actually you can get super depressed."[30]

Common symptoms of histamine intolerance include:[31]

> ➤ Headaches/migraines
> ➤ Difficulty falling asleep, easily aroused
> ➤ Hypertension
> ➤ Vertigo or dizziness

- ➢ Arrhythmia, or accelerated heart rate
- ➢ Difficulty regulating body temperature
- ➢ Anxiety
- ➢ Nausea, vomiting
- ➢ Abdominal cramps
- ➢ Flushing
- ➢ Nasal congestion, sneezing, difficulty breathing
- ➢ Abnormal menstrual cycle
- ➢ Hives
- ➢ Fatigue
- ➢ Tissue swelling

How do I break down histamine?

Once formed, histamine is either stored or broken down by an enzyme. Histamine in the central nervous system is broken down primarily by histamine N-methyltransferase (HMT), while histamine in the digestive tract is broken down primarily by diamine oxidase (DAO).

Though both enzymes play an important role in histamine breakdown, the American Society for Clinical Nutrition® found that DAO is the main enzyme responsible for breaking down ingested histamine. So if you're deficient in DAO, you likely have symptoms of histamine intolerance.[32]

So back to the symptoms - do you have MTHFR along with significant depression?

Let's say you're heterozygous for both MTHFR 1298 + MTHFR 677 (so you have one of each snps). If there is nothting further to test you might want to take folate/folic acid to help your methylation cycles and keep your homocysteine levels in optimal ranges, BUT this kind of treatment could make you more depressed/anxious or increase your risk for cancer.

Why?

FIRST - Defining Under- and Over- Methylators

Let's say your whole blood histamine level is 90 ng/ml (or high on whatever metric your lab uses). According to Dr William Walsh (in his bestselling book "Nutrient Power: Heal Your Biochemistry and Heal Your Brain" by William J. Walsh, PhD) an optimal histamine range is 40-70 ng/ml (some say 25-65 ng/ml - according to which lab you use), thereby classifying someone who's higher than 70 as an "Undermethylator".

An Undermethylator is intolerant to folate because it lowers serotonin even more, making them more depressed.

Methylfolate Causes Cancer?

There is a common misconception, however, that the mere presence of an MTHFR mutation is synonymous with a methylation defect. This is by no means necessarily the case, even if an individual is homozygous for the gene.

The presence of the defective gene does not necessarily translate into a functional defect. In fact, the recent widespread indiscriminate prescription of methylfolate to compensate for the genetic mutation is not only misguided, but can actually make people who are undermethylated not only feel much worse, but also increase their risk of developing cancer.[33]

So How Do You Figure This Out?

In order to determine the actual functional methylation status in the body, whole blood histamine must be measured. Histamine levels correlate with the functionality of the methylation process.

Histamine and methyl are inversely related to one another. That is to say, if whole blood histamine is low, the individual will be overmethylated and if it is high, they will be undermethylated.

The protocols to treat the two conditions are different.[34]

Note:

For whole blood histamine test accuracy please take no anti-histamines for two weeks prior to the testing.

So What Causes Histamine Intolerance?

Common causes include:[35]

➢ Inflammatory bowel diseases (or anything that causes damage to the enterocytes -the cells that line the gut).

➢ Celiac disease.

➢ Intestinal dysbiosis.

➢ Small Intestinal Bacterial Overgrowth (SIBO).

➢ Parasitic infections, like Giardia.

➢ Leaky gut or increase in intestinal permeability.

➢ Alcohol or other DAO inhibitors.

➢ Excess biogenic amines in diet.

➢ Medications that increase histamine.

➢ Food allergies.

➢ Genetic polymorphisms, like MTHFR and others that lower DAO, MAO, ALDH.

➢ Vitamin cofactor deficiencies - enzymes, like DAO and MAO rely on vitamin co-factors and deficiencies these can also cause abnormal enzyme activity.

Too Much Folate Causes Depression?

➢ A wide range of abnormal chemistries and behaviors were observed in the depressive population.

➢ 5 chemical classifications (phenotypes) were identified, representing 95% of depressives.

➢ Distinctive symptoms and traits were identified for each depression group.

Chemical Classification of Depression[36]

➢ 38% Undermethylation.

➢ 20% Folate Deficiency.

➢ 17% Copper Overload.

➢ 15% Elevated Pyrroles.

➢ 5% Toxic Metal Overload.

Implications of Database Findings on Depression[37]

➢ Depression is a name given to a variety of different mood disorders.

➢ Each depression phenotype has unique chemical imbalances and symptoms.

➢ Different treatment approaches are needed for these disorders.

A 25-Year Mystery Solved![38]

➢ Folate is a very-effective methylating agent.

➢ Undermethylated depressed patients (HIGH Histamine Level) are intolerant to folates.

➢ Overmethylated depressives (LOW Histamine Level) thrive on folates.

Serotonin Mystery Solved by Epigenetic Science[39]

➤ Folate generates acetylase enzymes that alter histones & promote expression of SERT (SERT = serotonin transporter).

➤ SERT increases serotonin reuptake, thus reducing serotonin activity.

➤ For low-serotonin depressives, the harmful impact of folic acid at the synapse exceeds the benefits of normalizing methylation.

Epigenetics of Methyl and Folate[40]

➤ SAMe modifies histones to block production of transporter proteins: This reuptake inhibition increases activity of serotonin & dopamine.

➤ Folates have the opposite effect on histones and lower serotonin and dopamine activity.

Facts About Methylation

Methylation is the act of a carbon and three hydrogens (namely a methyl group) attaching itself to an enzyme in your body. When this methyl group attaches to an enzyme, the enzyme performs a specific action.

One thing you might not realize is that methylation is responsible for the breakdown of histamine. A methyl group is made, and then floats around until it finds a specific binding site. In this case, the methyl group binds to histamine. When a methyl group binds to histamine, histamine breaks apart and goes away.

Many patients who have one or more methylation SNPs, like MTHFR, have a hard time breaking down histamine, which can wreak havoc on the body in many ways.[41]

IMPORTANT NOTE: When it comes to methylation - you either don't make enough, make too much, or make just the right amount. Be cautious with the use of folate/folic acid if you are an undermethylator. Folate is a serotonin reuptake promoter, (antidepressants [SSRI's] are reuptake inhibitors and undermethylated persons respond well to these medications) so its affect on your epigenetic structure will make you feel worse.

Plus, we already talked about this, just because you have the MTHFR genes, it does not mean that they are expressing. There are many epigentic reasons for turning them on and off.

In my opinion it would be very dangerous for anyone to tell a patient to take folate/folic acid if they don't know their methylation status (under-, normal, or over-).

Some symptoms and traits of undermethylation:[42]

Chronic depression, history of perfectionism, seasonal allergies, history of oppositional defiance, high libido, adverse reaction to benzodiazepines and folic acid, good response to SSRI's and anti-histamines, sparse body hair, suicidal tendencies, addictiveness, phobias, denial of illness, obsessive compulsive tendencies, ritualistic behaviors, strong willed, self-motivated during school years, history of competitiveness in sports, calm demeanor but high inner tension, family history of high accomplishment, frequent headaches, slenderness, dietary inflexibility, terse speech.

Some symptoms and traits of overmethylation:[43]

This is when your "METHYL WELL" is overflowing – this is bad – this is the crash you can expect as you get to where you need to be. Bumping up against these symptoms is inevitable. But informative too.

High anxiety/panic, hyperactivity, rapid speech, low libido, religiosity, tendency to be overweight, nervous legs, pacing, adverse reaction to SSRI's and SAMe, improvement with benzodiazepines, dry eyes and mouth, low motivation during school years, depression, self mutilation, sleep disorder, tinnitus, hirsutism, food/chemical sensitivities, increase artistic or musical ability, copper overload, estrogen and antihistamine intolerance, absence of seasonal allergies.

SAMe Supplementation – Is It Right?

Another aspect is that SAMe is great for an undermethylator but can cause suicidal/homicidal tendencies in an overmethylator because their serotonin levels are already elevated.

What if you have a "NORMAL Methylator"? Also it is possible that someone is a "normal" methylator and they would be in the range of 40-70 ng/ml (if your lab uses this range). Therefore, these normal methylator persons should be able to handle folate/folic acid. If someone is close to the edge of the range, either lower or upper ends of the range, then they would need to work with their doctor closely to see if they could tolerate folate (close to 70 range) or tolerate SAMe or methionine (close to the 40 range).

So you should incorporate whole blood histamine testing in your labs for your MTHFR testing.

Because then a "depressed person with MTHFR SNPs" wouldn't become more depressed by taking folate/folic acid and an overmethylator person with the MTHFR SNPs wouldn't become suicidal by mistakenly taking SAMe.

Someone who took SAMe

Let's look at a blog post by someone who took SAMe – THIS IS VERY INFORMATIVE.

BLOG POST FROM PGEN PARTICIPANT[44]

"Trying Out SAMe (Smart People Can Do Dumb Things)

First off, it turns out that methylfolate helps people make their OWN SAM-e! They are part of the same cycle, and SAM-e is one of the by-products from MTHFR processing. Regarding taking both, there was virtually no solid evidence floating up to the top, but an awful lot of opinion and personal experience. (Guess I'm adding to that body of unclear literature.) I saw a lot of people saying, "If you have MTHFR deficiency, do not ever take SAMe!" This was balanced by an equal number of folk saying the opposite. The overall picture was unclear. There was a lot that said to take them together, almost nothing about if you have an MTHFR deficiency.

I found one woman who described it as helpful for brief periods, and she described her genetics as similar to mine — heterozygous MTHFR, homozygous COMT (H62H & V158M), and celiac. She described reacting with an over-methylation response after a couple weeks, and I had gone through that when I started taking methylfolate and felt I know what to do. Just to be careful, I started out with the smallest dose I could find – 200mg.

WHAT HAPPENED

Part of what was motivating this was that general feeling of being unwell that I've had ever since I returned from my trip. I really want to feel better, but am feeling crummy. I thought about waiting to start SAMe until I feel better, but based on what information I'd found I thought I knew what to expect. Either it wouldn't do much, or I'd feel better.

I took a half dose on Monday. I felt basically the same as I've been feeling — generally crummy. Tuesday the same thing. I wasn't sure if I'd been glutened or not. I took a couple days off, just to see. Then I thought maybe I hadn't taken enough to notice a difference. [The problem with this was I had forgotten to look at how long it takes to feel an effect, and it varies depending on the problem.]

I was taking Friday as vacation, and thought I'd risk taking a larger dose, since I didn't want to experiment if I was going to try to work. Instead of 200, I took 400. I continued to feel vaguely crummy, and then I started to feel as if I'd been glutened. I'd been eating "whole foods," so I couldn't imagine what it would have been, but I recognized the feeling. Fatigue. Brain fog. Wobbly. But not a hint of any digestive symptoms, no bloating, no hives. I was puzzled, but sleeping too much to figure it out. I had trouble sitting and standing, my joints hurt. I felt too weak to do much. Not normal symptoms included feeling hot, sweaty, feverish, flushed, confused, congested, chilling, spaced out, distractible. Then I got a headache, and my head feels strange in the back. So far, this has lasted three days. Each day has had a couple brief periods when I felt ok, before it would start up again, slightly milder than the day before.

WHAT I LEARNED AFTERWARDS

I went back and looked again at SAMe overdose. Nope, these symptoms don't match up, except for the headache. My symptoms were more like those indicators that someone needs more SAMe. Very puzzling. I kept digging into literature about SAM-e. I tried taking extra methylfolate, but didn't notice a difference. I did notice that my clear-headed time was in late afternoon, and every day I take a B-complex vitamin with my lunch. Then I stumbled into some information that SAM-e can cause problems if someone is deficient in B-vitamins (like me). Basically, it creates a lot of homocysteine, which the body can't clear out because it needs more B-vitamins to do so."

Details: The Function Of SAMe

"What is the function of SAMe? The function of SAMe is to simply take what is called a 'methyl group' and give it away to over 200 enzymes in the body in order to perform various critical functions. Some key functions of this freely donated methyl group are to:

Protect your DNA. This is very important. For example, if your DNA is not protected, then it is susceptible to damage by viruses, bacteria, heavy metals, solvents and others. Over time, this damage becomes significant and may result in cancerous cell proliferation.

Reduce histamine levels! Repeat this so it sinks in. A methyl group given away by SAMe helps eliminate histamine from the body. Those with allergies or rashes may have higher levels of histamine and decreased methyl groups.

Produce a key component for your cell membranes called phosphatidylcholine. The methyl group donated by SAMe helps build phosphatidylcholine which then gets incorporated into the walls of all your cells, known as cell membranes. If these cell membranes become damaged and weak, the cells become fragile, allow toxins and harmful things into the cell, do not carry in useful nutrients, and then they die. Excessive cell membrane damage can lead to serious medical conditions, such as multiple sclerosis and cancer to name a few.[45]

SAMe[46]

SAMe is a naturally occurring metabolite found in the human body as well as in plant and animal foods. It is the most active of all methyl donors and has been compared to ATP in its importance for the body. SAMe is naturally synthesized in humans from the amino acid methionine in the presence of the cofactors B12 and folate.

SAMe is involved in the synthesis of neurotransmitters, the hormone melatonin, phospholipids, and polyamines, which control cellular growth. It is also the source of methyl groups inside the nucleus for DNA methylation, which controls gene expression and masking of genetic damage.

These capsules provide 200 mg of SAMe along with vitamins B6, B12, and folate as 5-MTHF, in order to provide cofactors for the natural conversions of SAMe to L-homocysteine and then safely to L-cysteine.

Plus, it's made with non-GMO ingredients.

CHAPTER SUMMARY

➤ First GET a WHOLE BLOOD HISTAMINE LEVEL – you need to know your status – have it drawn when they first check your Homocysteine level. REMEMBER - if Whole Blood Histamine is low, the individual will be overmethylated and if it is high, they will be undermethylated.

➤ Undermethylator (High Histamine Level >70 ng/ml) – SAMe works for these! However, try a methionine 500 mg caps or powder first. This should make them happy! But don't give folate/folic acid! Also antidepressant SSRIs tend to work well with these people.

➤ Overmethylator (Low Histamine Level <40 ng/ml) – SAMe makes patients suicidal – DO NOT GIVE! Give folate instead. Plus SSRIs are bad for these people. If the patient is depressed, use a TCA (tri-cyclic anti-depressant) such as low dose amitryptiline at night (25 mg).

12

NIACIN SUPPLEMENTATION FOR NAUSEA

What to Do If You Can't Tolerate ANY Methylfolate?

YUP – I'VE SEEN clients like this. They take the tiniest amount and spiral into depression or anxiety attacks or start to feel itchy. This is horrible – especially on a Friday afternoon or night! In this situation, it's tiny-dose niacin to the rescue (however, know occasionally it's tiny dose B6). For whatever reason, taking about 10-50 mg of niacin (though hard to find, 25 mg of niacin seems ideal) – this is usually 1/10th or even less of a 500 mg niacin tablet. It's a tiny dose, but for many people it really helps to ease the transition into taking methylfolate.[47] Some of my patients will take it every other day or some will take 4 every day, but they figure it out.

AUTHOR NOTE:

We use Niacin at 25 mg and have not yet had to use less than 10 mg.

A few days later, after the smoke has cleared, I have them take a dose of the methylfolate (methylfolate crumb?). Have them also take a tiny dose of niacin at the same time.

If niacin doesn't help, then sometimes hydroxycobalamin (B6) will. "This is a little bit mysterious because you'd think it would be methylcobalamin (the methylated form of B12 which MTHFR mutants also have a hard time making). Oddly, the hydroxycobalamin form seems to be the most helpful when you're starting L-5-MTHF dosing and when niacin doesn't take the edge off, a lot of times hydroxycobalamin will. Do you see what I mean about trial and error?"[48]

You can buy the niacin over the counter and use it accordingly.

13

GLUTATHIONE

MANY PEOPLE WITH MTHFR cannot make glutathione, especially the reduced version (GSH), so glutathione must be supplemented.

This is a bad thing as glutathione helps us detox (strongest anti-oxidant in the body), prevents heavy metal problems, and prevents toxin build-up. Lack of GSH (reduced glutathione) is the root cause of autism cases, and so forth.

Children on the Autism Spectrum Disorder (ASD) or even frank autism often can't make glutathione and so can't clear heavy metals (underlying hallmark of ASD). Pleas look at my #1 book on Amazon regarding Autism for more information (Natural Therapies for Autism: Updates on the Research By Dan Purser MD)

It's due to the inability to handle methionine or SAMe properly.

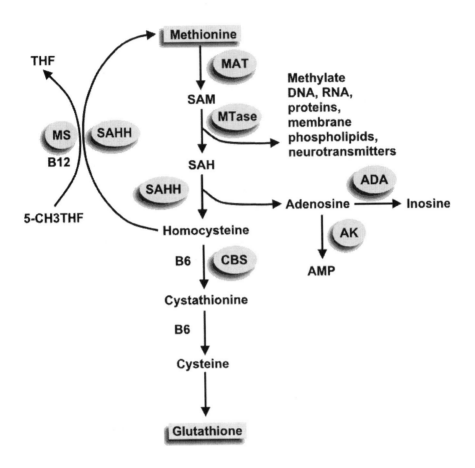

Without methionine you cannot make glutathione.

Period.

So these ASD and MTHFR patients tend to always have a shortage of glutathione on hand.

Facts Regarding Glutathione

The glutathione image has suffered from many problems – almost none of them really work – there is a lot if useless glutathione out there.

Why is this?

PROBLEM #1

Orals Digested In The Gut Do NOT Work.

Most are oral – when they hit the stomach they are all digested into their individual amino acids then broken down further as necessary. They are useless. Peer reviewed studies have shown these do not help in any way shape or form[49] [50].

So no "gut metabolized oral glutathione" will work (notice how I worded that).

Problem #2

What You Take Needs To Be Reduced Glutathione (Called GSH)

It's rarely a problem for anyone to make glutathione in their body (unless they have a cysteine deficiency – so remove this risk by taking n-acetyl-cysteine or NAC or better yet NACA[51]), but the problem is that most people with ASD or MTHFR cannot reduce glutathione back to its active form (GSH). This is probably the most common problem out there.

MOST PEOPLE WHO NEED GLUTATHIONE CAN MAKE IT THEY JUST CANNOT REDUCE IT BACK TO GSH.

"Reduced glutathione (Glutathione-SulfhHydryl or GSH) is a linear tripeptide of L-glutamine, L-cysteine, and glycine. Technically N-L-gamma-glutamyl-cysteinyl glycine or L-glutathione, the molecule has a sulfhydryl (SH) group on the cysteinyl portion, which accounts for its strong electron-donating character.

As electrons are lost, the molecule becomes oxidized, and two such molecules become linked (dimerized) by a disulfide bridge to form glutathione disulfide or oxidized glutathione (GSSG). This linkage is reversible upon re-reduction."[52]

GSH is under tight homeostatic control both intracellularly and extracellularly. A dynamic balance is maintained between GSH synthesis, its recycling from GSSG/oxidized glutathione, and its utilization. But it is this "re-reduction" that deficient people cannot perform.

So when you take it, if you need it, you must use the reduced or GSH form.

The problem with taking the reduced form or even finding it is that is almost always oxidized by air – even the intravenous forms (after 30 minutes or more). So the GSH must be protected – either complexed into a nano or lipodermal structure – but this requires a patented process that is only owned by one group of researchers – us (my team and friends).

So it cannot be swallowed orally, and it must be in the reduced (GSH) form protected by a nano or lipodermal structure.

Are there other problems?

PROBLEM #3

Carrier Must Be Stable

The carrier (nano sugar or the lipoderm) protects the GSH from air or other contaminants which would react with the GSH, oxidizing it. The carrier structure MUST be stable – since if it only lasts a few minutes or days it is worthless. Stable in the supplement world means for up to two (2) years. This is why we chose the nano carbohydrate striucture or the lipoderm – both work and stay (when in a cool oxygen free environment) stable indefinitely.

PROBLEM #4

If In A Nano Or Lipoderm Structure, The GSH Should Be Stored In An Airproof Container

This goes without saying, especially when considering the first THREE PROBLEMS, but it does not make it any easier – finding the right airproof container is very difficult. From this container you dispense the GSH.

Make sure the one you buy has this type of container.

PROBLEM #5

Is The GSH Concentrated Enough?

You must make sure you're getting an adequate dose. I would advise 500 mg/dose at least.

PROBLEM #6

The GSH Should Smell Like Rotten Eggs (Sulfhydryl Or Sulfur Smell)

The GSH you buy, if oral lipodermal (lipodermal GSH) if designed properly are transmucosal in their absorption and can be absorbed in your mouth and throat through the cells there. These should probably taste okay but should smell like rotten eggs.

Yuck!

I know. Hold your nose though and swallow. If the GSH or glutathione does not have this rotten egg odor, then it is not reduced, or active, or probably even real. It's that SH or sulfhydryl group that gives it this odor. Fake GSH will not have this smell, but I've found even top notch pharmacologists and big pharma execs do not know this (amazing as they turn up on our patented stable reduced GSH).

A nanoized (complexed to a carbohydrate) should also have the same smell if it's indeed reduced.

PROBLEM #7

Intravenous GSH IS Usually Oxidized By the Time You Are Given It

The GSH preparations used clinically by doctors for their patients in hospitals have a very short shelf life. It must be prepared by a compounding pharmacist daily, and used quickly, or all of the reduced, (active form) of the glutathione will be oxidized within an hour or less and be useless in most health care settings. So glutathione can be given intravenously but there are mixed results on the efficacy and/or practicality of this invasive therapy. Because of the above "time-sensitive-usage issue" and other problems, intravenous GSH is usually extraordinarily expensive and is used in very few institutions.

RULES

Lipodermal GSH (if the manufacturer guarantees reduced status and utilizes an airproof container or bottle) can be used either "swish-and-swallow-orally" or topically. You would absorb it either way (when you swish-and-swallow it would coat and absorb to the mucosa and then be absorbed through those cells).

Transmucosal delivery is not a new concept or a particularly difficult one. I pulled this off Google® Images™.

Transmucosal medication delivery

- Is this really a novel idea?
- Commercially available transmucosal drugs:
  - Actiq oral (transmucosal fentanyl lollipop)
  - Nitroglycerin – Sublingual.
  - Stadol (butorphanol) – Intranasal opiate.
  - Fentora – Transmucosal fentanyl tablet
  - DDAVP – Intranasal delivery route.
  - Migraine medications – Migranal (DHE), etc.
  - Influenza Vaccine – Intranasal system is available.
- Active area of pharmacology research

GSH has also been used in inhalation treatments in COPD patients with less than promising results. The fact that they are aerosolizing the GSH in a breathing treatment mixes the reduced GSH with its nemesis oxygen. This would instantly oxidize the GSH to GSSG and there would then be little if any benefit.

There has never before now been a good, inexpensive source of exogenous reduced GSH that could be used by, or readily available to the public. Which is too bad, because as we age we produce less GSH than we did when we were young and healthy.

GSH clearly is key to proper immune function. This is demonstrated by using the most extreme example available in our society today. AIDS patients, at the very end of their lives have serum GSH levels that are virtually undetectable. The concept of readily available exogenous GSH could possibly reduce the suffering and possibly extend the lives of those who are immune-compromised for any reason.

We are not making any claims that glutathione can cure AIDS (that would be crazy) but we believe that these patients would benefit from exogenous GSH supplementation. There are tens-of-thousands of articles on GSH in the medical literature. What is lacking are clinical trials on GSH because it is so unstable, expensive, and unavailable in most medical institutions. Our hope is that our product can start this road to discovery of new treatments and that others will join us in researching treatment possibilities.

It is well established that our bodies use endogenous GSH to keep our melanocytes from transitioning to melanomas.

Our livers use GSH to conjugate alcohol, acetaminophen and countless other electrophiles and/or toxins that could cause irreversible organ damage.

Heavy metals such as arsenic, lead, and mercury are removed from our bodies via GSH dependent mechanisms and pathways.

GSH and other antioxidants protect us from macular degeneration and macular dystrophy.

Accumulation of toxins and free-radicals cause damage that make us feel bad, make us look bad, and could be prevented.

GSH is vital for DNA repair and replication.

Low GSH levels have been associated with both hearing and visual impediments as we age.

Low GSH levels are observed in the pleural fluid of COPD patients, cystic fibrosis patients, and some forms of asthma.

GSH is vital for proper kidney function, proper liver function, proper lung function and proper immune function (including defense from cold and flu).

Accumulation of excess oxygen and nitrogen free-radicals formed by normal muscle contraction cause a decrease in muscle force production and premature muscle fatigue.

There are NO antioxidants known that are as efficient or efficacious as GSH in neutralizing free radicals and generally cleaning up the internal mess we sometimes make, (i.e., breathing smog, smoking, eating things we shouldn't, drinking things we shouldn't, exposing our fragile skin to UV-rays, and every variety of topical insults we expose ourselves to).

Other antioxidants are often rated by comparing themselves to GSH and claiming they are some percentage as good as GSH. Nothing even comes close, and many antioxidants require GSH to work properly.

GSH is vital for so many physiologic and protective functions that this book was written to begin the discussion of uses and benefits of exogenous GSH therapy. Because there's never before been available an actual working exogenous form of stable absorbable GSH, this discussion is just beginning.

People who supplement GSH by ingesting precursors of glutathione claim increased energy, a general feeling of well-being, reduced fatigue, weight loss, increased mental clarity and ability to focus and stay on task, increased energy, increased libido and so many other positive reactions that we feel we must revisit these benefits later in this book.

A topical GSH supplement may provide these same benefits and more. Again, we make no claims at this point. All discussion in this book refers to GSH in general terms.

There has been much discussion in our circles as to what actually is GSH. To be true to my scientific roots I insist that it is not a vitamin. It is not a mineral. It is not a hormone. It is not really a protein. It is not a lipid. It is not a carbohydrate. It is not a food. It is not a by-product. It is not an enzyme. It is not a co-enzyme. It is not a precursor to a more important compound. It is not a "cure-all". It is not "snake-oil". It is not a cucumber, (perhaps I go too far...). The others I work with hate when I say the following... but here it is.

"Glutathione is a ubiquitous, endogenous low-molecular-weight thiol tripeptide"

This is the best description of what GSH actually is.

Having listed what GSH is not, here is what we know that it is, (this list will undoubtedly grow as we learn more).

GSH is a tripeptide made up of three amino acids, (glutamate, glycine and the key amino acid that has the highly reactive sulfur group... cysteine).

GSH is the most powerful antioxidant known to science. It can serve as a modulator and in signaling roles in physiological processes. It is made in certain cells types in our bodies and can be exported by these cells to areas that require higher GSH concentrations or to cells that do not make their own GSH, (ie. glial cells in the brain make and recycle GSH, while neurons and astrocytes do not).

The brain uses more oxygen by weight than any other tissue or organ system. This oxygen is used with glucose to make ATP in the mitochondria of the cells via the electron transport chain (ETC - which ends with CoQ10 – something we discuss later). Oxygen free radicals leak from the electron transport chain and cause problems. Neurons, astrocytes and other nervous system cells are protected by the GSH made in glial cells and exported to where it is needed. Simple, right?

What do you suppose happens if you are not making enough GSH and the free-radicals and other toxins build up? It might explain why you feel groggy and sluggish at work in the afternoon. Your body wants you to rest and sleep so these insults can be cleared and GSH levels have enough time to normalize.

GSH is formed in our bodies using specific enzyme pathways. It is recycled between reduced state, (GSH) and oxidized state, (GSSG) by other enzymatic pathways, (that is if we are young and healthy). Its production in our bodies decreases with age, as much as 10-15% per decade after age 20, or even more quickly with trauma or other illnesses. There are many, many other things that GSH "is" and that it does.

Why do I tell you all this? Why tell you about the complexed GSH? Because I am not convinced NAC (n-acetyl-cysteine) alone can increase glutathione levels in someone with enzymatic problems such as MTHFR deficient individuals, or children with ASD (who also have MTHFR enzyme deficiency). Topical non-digestible, reduced, absorbable, stable GSH (glutathione) may be the only viable option. That's why...

14

HOMOZYGOUS C677T THERAPY

THIS IS A real problem – if this is the result of your genetic testing then you are in for it (you almost assuredly already realize this), so this approach must be handled very carefully.

Note that having just one C677T snp (technically *Heterozygous C677T*) can possibly give you up to a 40% decline MTHFR enzyme functionality – please look at the results of Patient 3 - the Spectracell® Comprehensive Micronutrient Panel, and the Spectracell® MTHFR Genetic test also. You'd treat this the same way as a Homozygous C677T recipient.

I am going to give you my approach to this – but please look at Dr. Ben Lynch's protocol on his website – it is an incredibly detailed and micromanaged approach from MTHFR.net – you definitely need to go to the website and review it.

Dan Purser M.D. – My Take On HOMOZYGOUS C677T THERAPY

Homozygous C677T mutations can either be:

1) The hard tip of a HUGE genetic iceberg of errors (most of us tend to have hundreds) that has wiped out all kinds of enzymes and caused all kinds of problems or,

2) Can be "just" a severe stand-alone MTHFR problem (less likely).

Your parents had some idea as you started to mature that something was off – you complained of being tired all the time, and maybe were sad a lot, and in sports you could not keep up with the other kids, no matter how hard you tried.

Though they did not know this and could not see this, the severe "iceberg" carried with it a myriad of other gene mutations affecting innumerable enzymes which could cause mental and neurological developmental difficulties with all kinds of developmental challenges, OR:

You seemed completely normal (other than never being able to keep up and being tired when compared to other children, except now you realize you never really felt normal).

As a medical practitioner I need to assume patients fall somewhere in between the two, and so I feel like I have to dive fairly deep here. Once I realize you're genetically homozygous C677T, then I will suggest a couple of other labs that need to be sorted out – a Homocysteine level, a whole blood histamine level, and a Spectracell™ (intracellular) Comprehensive Micronutrient Panel (since this test, among many other things, will show intracellular B6 and zinc levels) you need to get a urinary pyrrole level – it's redundant. If the intracellular zinc and B6 levels are low, then they are more than likely being pulled into the urine (by excess pyrroles) and flushed away. These tests are all drawn because I'm looking for additional enzyme defects or gene mutations that are occurring concurrently with the C677T (more of the iceberg beneath the water type of thing).

Just to be safe, I would use a tiny dose of folate (200 mcg or less) or even folinic acid (more natural) to begin with. Maybe in the form of a whole food multivitamin as its dose of natural folate seems to be the BEST starting product on the market for MTHFR, especially for Homozygous C677T condition. But another option is to start on Folinic Acid 500 mcg (try half of one of whatever size you can find) or B12 500 mcg (even try half of one per day – but whichever path you choose, start low and go slow!

Then after a few weeks I'd switch to that main "methylation support" you found -- and a conservative approach (which I would advise) would be to start on one a day – then go to two a day, then more as needed – maybe as many as 8/day at the doses I recommended. The reason I conclude this is from experience.

WARNING!

You have to realize there is a problem that can occur as you slowly increase the amount of the main "methylation support" – you might overcome the methylation capabilities. This will cause achiness and flu-like symptoms -- these symptoms can be severe, and usually occur a few days after a step up in dosage (from say 5/day to 6/day as an example) – when this happens you must stop the "methylation support" for a day or two, and go back to the last dose that was comfortable. In a few months or weeks, you can try going up again.

Make sure you temporarily stop the folate and multivitamin when you start on the "methylation support" – one in the morning when you first wake up. If you have no problems, then slowly going up each week until you are on 2 in the morning then later you can try adding up to 2 before lunch, and then eventually up to 8/day in divided doses – that's the about the maximum dose. This is not my approach originally but borrowed from Dr. Ben Lynch at MTHFR.net who suggests this step-wise approach.

All this should bring down the Homocysteine level to normal (check every few months until down to normal – then every 6-12 months thereafter).

Before going further along this path, you must determine the methylation status, and this status is determined by the whole blood histamine level.

Why the Whole Blood Histamine level?

It is so difficult to determine methylation capabilities in every human, even if you know their MTHFR gene status – that knowledge is just not enough. We do not know the complexity of the effects of the genetic errors (I say "we just don't know what lies beneath") that are also causing problems (remember that we all have dozens if not hundreds of these genetic errors and mutations). This makes trying to guess on methylation status basically impossible without getting a whole blood histamine level.

Remember:

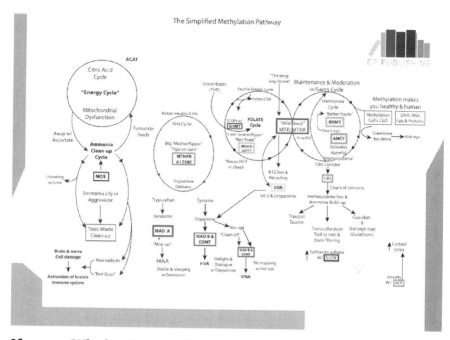

The Simplified Methylation Pathway

If your Whole Blood Histamine is greater than > 65-70 ng/ml (or HIGH) then you are an "UNDERMETHYLATOR" (38%) and you should AVOID EXCESS FOLATE (which would cause depression to occur or worsen) and take SAMe. If you don't do this you might have depression.

If your Whole Blood Histamine is less than > 25-40 ng/ml (LOW) then you are an "OVERMETHYLATOR" and you should avoid and take folate. Lack of this could cause anxiety.

NOTE:

HIGH is "UNDER--"
LOW is "OVER –"METHYLATOR

Some patients will have nausea or anxiety as their dose of "methylation support" climbs – what do you take for this nausea or anxiety? Add Niacin 25 mg – add just one and see how you do. You may need more than one – you can take up to 6-10 but usually one or two is enough.

GUT PROBLEMS? Common with this condition. I use probiotics – it's the best option. B6 (25 mg/day) and Zinc (50 mg/day) along with the probiotics may help. See my Amazon™ book on Copper Toxicity XXXXX for more possible assistance in this area.

So here is the protocol:

HOMOZYGOUS C677T PROTOCOL© BY DAN PURSER M.D.

1. Get your SpectraCell© Comprehensive Micronutrient Panel - critical, and saves a ton of money on enzyme testing.

2. Get Your Whole Blood Histamine Level – helps determine methylation status.

3. Get your Homocysteine Level – determines inflammation status and treatment value.

4. Start with a natural whole food multivitamin at one per day (one capsule or tablet or packet, if chosen correctly, is the easiest and most natural way to get a TINY AMOUNT OF NATURAL FOLATE IN).

5. Add fish oil – no matter what the front of the bottle says, your goal is to get 2500 mg/day of EPA and DHA – start with one per day (with meals) and after a few weeks go to twice a day (to prevent clotting, strokes, and other thrombotic events).

6. Add probiotics -- 2 in the morning or two at night – take with food.

7. If you have any clotting risk (check with your doctor) add nattokinase (2,000 Fu), to reduce clotting risk naturally.

8. After 1-2 weeks, if you have no nausea, add or start on Folic Acid 500 mcg (try half of one per day).

9. After two weeks with no problems (nausea, aches, pains, etc.) add your chosen "methylation support" capsule as I outlined at one per day. Take it first thing in the morning.

10. After one week increase the "methylation support" capsule to two per day.

11. After another week and no problems (i.e. flu-like symptoms), go to three per day (2 in AM and 1 at lunch).

12. Nauseated or feel funky? Add NIACIN at 25 mg a dose (watch for flushing – just a weird side effect). Take up to 6 per day (they're safe but you just may flush which can be misery).

13. Is your Whole Blood Histamine level **high**? You are an "**undermethylator**". Start with methionine 200 or 250 mg capsules first. If two each day are well tolerated, then change to SAMe (and avoid extra methylfolate or especially folic acid!).

14. Is your Whole Blood Histamine level **low**? You are an "**overmethylator**". Then add B12 500 mcg, slowly climbing to 1-3 per day – but do it SLOWLY.

15. After a few weeks and feeling the benefits (you will), please take an extra "methylation support" capsule at noon, before lunch, or with lunch (so now you're on 4/day).

16. After a few more weeks try 5 "methylation support" capsules per day (3 in AM and 2 at lunch). If you have

nausea or flu-like problems, back it back down to three or four per day.

17. Keep going up on the "methylation support" capsule until you hit 8. That will be your dose. Forever.

18. WARNING! If you ever miss or stop taking your "methylation support" capsule you will probably feel pretty horrible pretty quickly (a day or two into it?). If you don't believe try it and see for your self. You crash back to how you used to feel pretty fast. It is not good. DO NOT STOP your "methylation support" capsule.

19. Add other vitamins as needed according to the SpectraCell® Results.

20. Don't forget to add Niacin (25 mg) or B6 (25 mg -- in the form of hydroxycobalamin) if nausea occurs.

21. What should you feel now? Welcome to normalcy. You should feel TONS of ENERGY. Your testosterone or other hormones (unless you're in menopause) should be slowly rising after 3-4 months – eventually to a much more normal level. It becomes very obvious if we dialed it all in correctly. This approach should work for about 90% of C677T people, but for some it will not – so see your doctor or naturopath if it does not.

22. If you're in the 10% who do not feel better, be patient. Look to see if you're an under or over-methylator. See if you need methionine first, then try SAMe. Also, if you're anxious try GABA (500-600 mg at night) or 5-HTP to help you sleep. Or try TMG too. See if that helps. You have many options. DO NOT GIVE UP!

HOMOZYGOUS C677T PATIENT EXAMPLES

Patient 1: I got this Spectracell® first, and it made me go huh?

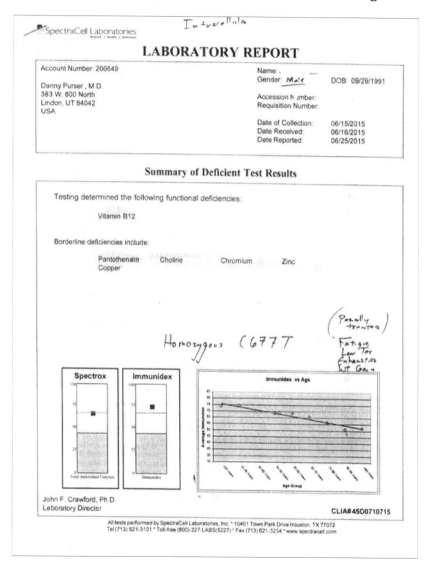

The genetic testing I ordered afterward – confirming my suspicions.

SpectraCell Laboratories

Science • Health • Solutions
10401 Town Park Drive
Houston, TX 77072

Phone: (713)621-3101
TollFree: (800)227-LABS(5227)
Fax: (281)568-5246

Laboratory Report

Account Number: 206649	Name:
	Gender: DOB: 9/29/1991
Danny Purser , M.D.	Accession Number:
383 W. 600 North	Requisition Number:
	Date Collected: June 15, 2015
Lindon, UT 84042	Date Received: June 16, 2015
	Date Reported: June 22, 2015

MTHFR Genotype Test Result

Test	Result
C677T Mutation	Homozygous
A1298C Mutation	Negative

This sample has two copies of the C677T mutation and is negative for the A1298C mutation.
This genotype

- is associated with decreased enzyme activity (approximately 30% of normal activity).
- is associated with increased homocysteine levels.
- is correlated with increased risk of cardiovascular disease or thrombosis.
- is associated with potential methotrexate intolerance and patients may require dosage adjustments or
  discontinuation.

John F. Crawford, Ph.D.
Laboratory Director

CLIA# 45D0710715

MTHFR Background Information

MTHFR (methylenetetrahydrofolate reductase) is an enzyme involved in the metabolism of folate and homocysteine. It plays a role in maintaining cellular folate levels and is a cofactor needed to convert homocysteine (a potentially toxic amino acid) to methionine.

Certain common genetic point mutations have been characterized that reduce the function of the MTHFR enzyme. These are the C677T mutation (which is a change from cytosine to thymine at position 677 within the gene) and the A1298C mutation (which is a change from adenine to cytosine at position 1298 within the gene.) An MTHFR enzyme with reduced function can lead to elevated homocysteine levels, which is a known independent risk factor for development of cardiovascular disease and venous thrombosis. Reduced enzyme function can also affect folate status.

An additional area in which the function of MTHFR can have an effect is during methotrexate therapy. Methotrexate is a drug often used in treatment of certain cancers or autoimmune diseases. It is a structural analogue of folate and can interfere with folate metabolism. Defects in folate metabolism such as those potentially arising from mutations affecting MTHFR function can increase sensitivity to methotrexate and may lead to lower dosage requirements, increased side effects, or intolerance of the drug.

Testing Limitations

Only the C667T and A1298C mutations are analyzed in this assay. There may be other unknown non-genetic factors or genetic factors besides the tested mutations that can affect homocysteine levels, folate status, or drug sensitivities. Rare mutations in the primer binding sites used to detect the C677T and A1298C mutations may prevent detection. Specific dosing guidelines for methotrexate based on MTHFR genotype are not currently available.

MTHFR genotyping can provide useful information concerning risks of developing cardiovascular disease or thrombosis, or potential for increased sensitivity to methotrexate treatment. However, genotyping alone is not predictive of development of disease or complication and should not be used as the primary means of clinical diagnosis or treatment decision making. This information should be used by a physician in conjunction with additional clinical information to determine an appropriate treatment regimen.

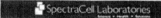
SpectraCell Laboratories

The vitamin page on the Spectracell® Metabolic Panel. Remember these values are intracellular.

ctraCell Laboratories, Inc.
aboratory Test Report

Accession Number:

Micronutrients	Patient Results (% Control)	Functional Abnormals	Reference Range (greater than)
B Complex Vitamins			
Vitamin B1 (Thiamin)	98		>78%
Vitamin B2 (Riboflavin)	73		>53%
Vitamin B3 (Niacinamide)	91		>80%
Vitamin B6 (Pyridoxine)	69		>54%
Vitamin B12 (Cobalamin)	14	Deficient	>14%
Folate	46		>32%
Pantothenate	9	Borderline	>7%
Biotin	43		>34%
Amino Acids			
Serine	53		>30%
Glutamine	52		>37%
Asparagine	54		>39%
Metabolites			
Choline	23	Borderline	>20%
Inositol	76		>58%
Carnitine	60		>46%
Fatty Acids			
Oleic Acid	71		>65%
Other Vitamins			
Vitamin D3 (Cholecalciferol)	58		>50%
Vitamin A (Retinol)	83		>70%
Vitamin K2	51		>30%
Minerals			
Calcium	44		>38%
Manganese	65		>50%
Zinc	42	Borderline	>37%
Copper	44	Borderline	>42%
Magnesium	45		>37%
Carbohydrate Metabolism			
Glucose-Insulin Interaction	57		>38%
Fructose Sensitivity	52		>34%
Chromium	44	Borderline	>40%
Antioxidants			
Glutathione	55		>42%
Cysteine	54		>41%
Coenzyme Q-10	92		>86%
Selenium	83		>74%
Vitamin E (A-tocopherol)	91		>84%
Alpha Lipoic Acid	90		>81%
Vitamin C	53		>40%
SPECTROX™			
Total Antioxidant Function	66		>40%
Proliferation Index			
Immunidex	71		>40%

The reference ranges listed in the above table are valid for male and female patients 12 years of age or older.

Patient 2 *Again I started with a Spectracell® due to the fatigue complaint.*

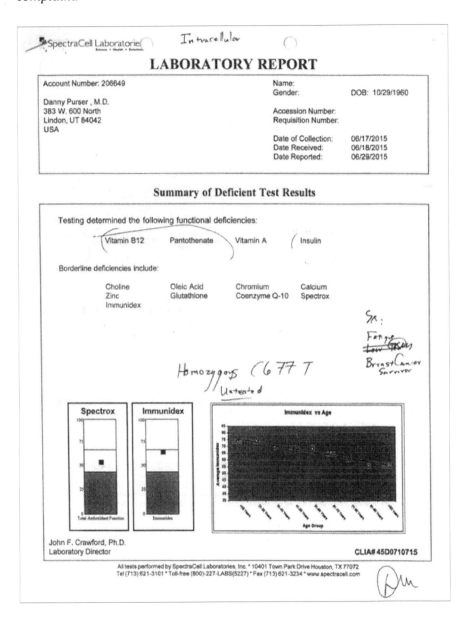

Micronutrients	Patient Results (% Control)	Functional Abnormals	Reference Range (greater than)
B Complex Vitamins			
Vitamin B1 (Thiamin)	97		>78%
Vitamin B2 (Riboflavin)	59		>53%
Vitamin B3 (Niacinamide)	99		>80%
Vitamin B6 (Pyridoxine)	60		>54%
Vitamin B12 (Cobalamin)	14	Deficient	>14%
Folate	42		>32%
Pantothenate	7	Deficient	>7%
Biotin	44		>34%
Amino Acids			
Serine	36		>30%
Glutamine	58		>37%
Asparagine	47		>39%
Metabolites			
Choline	22	Borderline	>20%
Inositol	72		>58%
Carnitine	63		>46%
Fatty Acids			
Oleic Acid	70	Borderline	>65%
Other Vitamins			
Vitamin D3 (Cholecalciferol)	59		>50%
Vitamin A (Retinol)	68	Deficient	>70%
Vitamin K2	69		>30%
Minerals			
Calcium	42	Borderline	>38%
Manganese	65		>50%
Zinc	42	Borderline	>37%
Copper	55		>42%
Magnesium	45		>37%
Carbohydrate Metabolism			
Glucose-Insulin Interaction	35	Deficient	>38%
Fructose Sensitivity	53		>34%
Chromium	41	Borderline	>40%
Antioxidants			
Glutathione	44	Borderline	>42%
Cysteine	54		>41%
Coenzyme Q-10	89	Borderline	>86%
Selenium	79		>74%
Vitamin E (A-tocopherol)	92		>84%
Alpha Lipoic Acid	88		>81%
Vitamin C	58		>40%
SPECTROX™			
Total Antioxidant Function	54	Borderline	>40%
Proliferation Index			
Immunidex	62	Borderline	>40%

The reference ranges listed in the above table are valid for male and female patients 12 years of age or older.

SpectraCell Laboratories
Science • Health • Solutions

Phone:	(713)621-3101
Toll Free:	(800)227-LABS(5227)
Fax:	(281)568-5246

Laboratory Report

Account Number:	206649	Name:	
		Gender:	DOB: 10/29/1960
Danny Purser , M.D.		Accession Number:	
383 W. 600 North		Requisition Number:	
Lindon, UT 84042			
USA		Date Collected:	July 15, 2015
(801) 785 8826		Date Received:	July 16, 2015
		Date Reported:	July 22, 2015

MTHFR Genotype Test Result

Test	Result
C677T Mutation	Homozygous
A1298C Mutation	Negative

This sample has two copies of the C677T mutation and is negative for the A1298C mutation. This genotype

• is associated with decreased enzyme activity (approximately 30% of normal activity).
• is associated with increased homocysteine levels.
• is correlated with increased risk of cardiovascular disease or thrombosis.
• is associated with potential methotrexate intolerance and patients may require dosage adjustments or discontinuation.

10401 Town Park Drive, Houston, Texas 77072 USA
(800)227-LABS(5227) / (713)-621-3101

CLIA# 45D0710715
J.F. Crawford, Ph.D., Laboratory Director

MTHFR Background Information

MTHFR (methylenetetrahydrofolate reductase) is an enzyme involved in the metabolism of folate and homocysteine. It plays a role in maintaining cellular folate levels and is a cofactor needed to convert homocysteine (a potentially toxic amino acid) to methionine.

Certain common genetic point mutations have been characterized that reduce the function of the MTHFR enzyme. These are the C677T mutation (which is a change from cytosine to thymine at position 677 within the gene) and the A1298C mutation (which is a change from adenine to cytosine at position 1298 within the gene.) An MTHFR enzyme with reduced function can lead to elevated homocysteine levels, which is a known independent risk factor for development of cardiovascular disease and venous thrombosis. Reduced enzyme function can also affect folate status.

An additional area in which the function of MTHFR can have an effect is during methotrexate therapy. Methotrexate is a drug often used in treatment of certain cancers or autoimmune diseases. It is a structural analogue of folate and can interfere with folate metabolism. Defects in folate metabolism such as those potentially arising from mutations affecting MTHFR function can increase sensitivity to methotrexate and may lead to lower dosage requirements, increased side effects, or intolerance of the drug.

Testing Limitations

Only the C667T and A1298C mutations are analyzed in this assay. There may be other unknown non-genetic factors or genetic factors besides the tested mutations that can affect homocysteine levels, folate status, or drug sensitivities. Rare mutations in the primer binding sites used to detect the C677T and A1298C mutations may prevent detection. Specific dosing guidelines for methotrexate based on MTHFR genotype are not currently available.

MTHFR genotyping can provide useful information concerning risks of developing cardiovascular disease or thrombosis, or potential for increased sensitivity to methotrexate treatment. However, genotyping alone is not predictive of development of disease or complication and should not be used as the primary means of clinical diagnosis or treatment decision making. This information should be used by a physician in conjunction with additional clinical information to determine an appropriate treatment regimen.

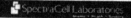

Visit us at www.spectracell.com or call us at 800.227.LABS (5227)

SpectraCell Laboratories

UH OH, THE MTHFR WOMAN IS AN "UNDERMETHYLATOR"

She quietly sat across from me as I explained her whole blood histamine level. Her homocysteine level was fine – not high, but I had started her on Powerful Mind™ before we did that test so maybe it had been high? But it was normal now.

It was her whole blood histamine level that had blown through the roof – it was really high. She was an undermethylator – meaning she probably had difficulty handling folates.

"You need to stop the Powerful Mind™ or at least hold your dose increases – maybe just take one a day."

"Why?"

"You're an undermethylator which means you can't tolerate lots of folate. You need methionine or SAMe instead. Because of your genetic errors, folate will decrease your serotonin causing you to be really tired or depressed – so that's why I am cutting back on your Powerful Mind™. The good news is SSRIs like Prozac™ can be very appropriate for you and help a lot. But let's try to get you a natural high."

"Does that mean vitamins won't work for me?"

"No, methionine will. So will SAMe. You just have to be *very careful* with folate. But we'll start you on the amino acid methionine first. 500 mg."

She nodded studying the bottle of methionine I had handed her.

When you get to two of those each morning with your Powerful Mind™, then we'll change it to some SAMe."

"What's this one going to make me feel like?"

"Happier. More upbeat and more energy. If not, then just stop the Powerful Mind completely and use the methionine or SAMe by themselves."

I slid her a bottle of SAMe that I liked.

"Well, at least you're trying to deal with the root cause."

I reassured her. "We'll get there."

She smiled and got up to leave.

I smiled.

15

IS THERE AN MTHFR DIET?

As I said earlier one version would be:

Methionine or Meat Restricted Diets

Methionine restriction is recommended for risk variant carriers to reduce homocysteine accumulation and limit the effects of reduced MTHFR activity. Since dietary methionine is mostly found in animal proteins, and folate is mainly found in vegetables, methionine restriction calls for vegetarian-orientated diets.

In vegetarian diet regimens, a vitamin B12 supplement is strongly recommended since it is primarily found in animal products.[53]

I also need to point out that the Dean Ornish SPECTRUM™ lifestyle diet is low in methionine and could be helpful too. His book can be purchased on Amazon®.

Many MTHFR experts[54] suggest this next diet as being the best for MTHFR. I said huh? So I wrote a cookbook for MTHFR – here it is: <u>MTHFR COOKBOOK & MEAL PLANS by Dan PurserMD</u>

Short of buying my cookbook here are some ideas.

RECOMMENDED FOODS

Almonds, including almond butter and oil

Apples

Apricots, fresh or dried

Artichoke

Asiago cheese

Asparagus

Aubergine (eggplant)

Avocados, including avocado oil

Bananas (ripe only with brown spots on the skin)

Beans, dried white (navy), string beans and lima beans

Beef, fresh or frozen

Beets or beetroot

Berries, all kinds

Black, white and red pepper: ground and pepper corns

Black radish

Blue cheese

Bok Choy

Brazil nuts

Brick cheese

Brie cheese

Broccoli

Brussels sprouts

Butter

Cabbage

Camembert cheese

Canned fish in oil or water only

Capers

Carrots

Cashew nuts, fresh only

Cauliflower

Cayenne pepper

Celeriac

Celery

Cellulose in supplements

Cheddar cheese

Cherimoya (custard apple or sharifa)

Cherries

Chicken, fresh or frozen

Cinnamon

Citric acid

Coconut, fresh or dried (shredded) without any additives

Coconut milk

Coconut oil

Coffee, weak and freshly made, not instant

Collard greens

Colby cheese

Courgette (zucchini)

Coriander, fresh or dried

Cucumber

Dates, fresh or dried without any additives (not soaked in syrup)

Dill, fresh or dried

Duck, fresh or frozen

Edam cheese

Eggplant

Eggs, fresh

Filberts

Fish, fresh or frozen

Game, fresh or frozen

Garlic

Ghee, homemade (many store varieties contain non-allowed ingredients)

Gin, occasionally

Ginger root, fresh

Goose, fresh or frozen

Gorgonzola cheese

Gouda cheese

Grapefruit

Grapes

Haricot beans

Havarti cheese

Hazelnuts

Herbal teas

Herbs, fresh or dried without additives

Honey, natural

Juices freshly pressed from permitted fruit and vegetables

Kale

Kiwi fruit

Kumquats

Lamb, fresh or frozen

Lemons

Lentils

Lettuce, all kinds

Lima beans (dried and fresh)

Limburger cheese

Limes

Mangoes

Melons

Monterey (Jack) cheese

Muenster cheese

Mushrooms

Mustard seeds, pure powder and gourmet types

Nectarines

Nut flour or ground nuts (usually ground blanched almonds)

Nutmeg

Nuts, all kinds freshly shelled, salted or coated (any roasting must be done at home)

Olive oil, virgin cold-pressed

Olives preserved without sugar

Onions

Oranges

Papayas

Parmesan cheese

Parsley

Peaches

Peanut butter, without additives

Peanuts, fresh or roasted in their shells at home

Pears

Peas, dried split and fresh green

Pecans

Peppers (green, yellow, red, and orange)

Pheasant, fresh or frozen

Pickles, without sugar

Pigeon, fresh or frozen

Pineapples, fresh

Pork, fresh or frozen

Port du Salut cheese

Poultry, fresh or frozen

Prunes, dried without any additives or in their own juice

Pumpkin

Quail, fresh or frozen

Raisins

Rhubarb

Roquefort cheese

Romano cheese

Satsumas

Scotch, occasionally

Seaweed fresh and dried

Shellfish, fresh or frozen

Spices, single and pure without any additives

Spinach

Squash (summer and winter)

Stilton cheese

String beans

Swedes

Swiss cheese

Tangerines

Tea, weak, freshly made, not instant

Tomato puree, pure without any additives apart from salt

Tomato juice, without any additives apart from salt

Tomatoes

Turkey, fresh or frozen

Turnips

Ugly fruit

Uncreamed cottage cheese (dry curd)

Vinegar (cider or white)

Vodka, very occasionally

Walnuts

Watercress

White navy beans

Wine: red or white

Yogurt, homemade

Zucchini (courgette)

****FOODS TO AVOID***

Acesulphame

Acidophilus milk

Agar-agar

Agave syrup - main carbohydrate is a complex form of fructose

Algae - can aggravate an already disturbed immune system

Aloe Vera - please go to "FAQs" for additional information on when it can be introduced

Amaranth - is a grain substitute, contains starches

Apple juice - usually has sugar added during processing

Arrowroot - is a mucilaginous herb and loaded with starch

Aspartame

Astragalus - contains polysaccharides

Baked beans

Baker's yeast - contains saccharamyces cerevisae

Baking powder and raising agents of all kind - baking soda can be used for specific medical issues, please view the "FAQs" section

Balsamic vinegar - most found in stores have added sugar

Barley

Bean flour and sprouts

Bee pollen - irritating to a damaged gut

Beer

Bhindi or okra

Bicarbonate of soda

Bitter Gourd

Black-eye beans

Bologna

Bouillon cubes or granules

Brandy

Buckwheat

Bulgur

Burdock root - contains FOS and mucilage

Butter beans

Buttermilk

Canellini beans

Canned vegetables and fruit

Carob

Cellulose gum

Cereals, including all breakfast cereals

Cheeses, processed and cheese spreads

Chestnuts and chestnut flour

Chevre cheese

Chewing gum - contain sugars or sugar substitutes

Chick peas

Chickory root - contains high amounts of FOS

Chocolate

Cocoa powder - please see "FAQs" for more information

Coffee, instant and coffee substitutes

Cooking oils

Cordials

Corn

Cornstarch

Corn syrup

Cottage cheese

Cottonseed

Cous-cous

Cream - contains lactose

Cream of Tartar

Cream cheese

Dextrose - in commercial products it is not the pure form

Faba beans

Feta cheese

Fish, preserved, smoked, salted, breaded and canned with sauces

Flour, made out of grains

FOS (fructooligosaccharides)

Fructose - extracted from corn and has a mixture of other trisaccharides

Fruit, canned or preserved

Garbanzo beans

Gjetost cheese

Grains, all

Gruyere cheese

Ham

Hot dogs

Ice-cream, commercial

Jams

Jellies

Jerusalem artichoke (also called sunroot or sunchoke)

Ketchup, commercially available

Lactose

Liqueurs

Margarines and butter replacements

Meats, processed, preserved, smoked and salted

Millet

Milk from any animal, soy, rice, canned coconut milk

Milk, dried

Molasses

Mozzarella cheese

Mungbeans

Neufchatel cheese

Nutra-sweet® (aspartame)

Oats

Okra - mucilaginous food

Parsnips

Pasta, of any kind

Pectin

Postum

Potato, white

Potato, sweet

Primost cheese

Quinoa - 60% starch

Rice

Ricotta cheese

Rye

Saccharin

Sago

Sausages, commercially available

Semolina

Sherry

Soda, soft drinks

Sour cream, commercial

Soy

Spelt

Starch

Sugar or sucrose of any kind

Tapioca - starch

Tea, instant

Triticale

Turkey loaf

Vegetables, canned or preserved

Wheat

Wheat germ

Whey, powder or liquid

Yams

Yogurt, commercial

For A1298C Homozygous – HIGH purine food diets help.
FOODS HIGH IN PURINES

The impact of plant purines on gout risk is very different from the impact of animal purines, and that within the animal food family, purines from meat and fish act very differently than purines from dairy.

EAT THESE —> Foods with high and moderately high purine levels (5-100 mg per 3.5 ounce serving):

Asparagus, Bacon, Beef, Bluefish, Bouillon, Calf tongue, Carp, Cauliflower, Chicken, Chicken soup, Codfish, Crab, Duck, Goose, Halibut, Ham, Kidney beans, Lamb, Lentils, Lima beans, Lobster, Mushrooms, Mutton, Navy beans, Oatmeal, Oysters, Peas, Perch, Pork, Rabbit, Salmon, Sheep, Shellfish, Snapper, Spinach, Tripe, Trout, Tuna, Turkey, Veal, Venison.[55]

RARELY EAT THESE —> Foods with very high purine levels (up to 1,000 mg per 3.5 ounce serving):

Anchovies, Grains, Gravies, Kidneys, Liver, Sardines, Sweetbreads[56]

(Look for my book on MTHFR Whole Blood Cookbook & Meal Plans   found   at   http://goo.gl/vwHg3K)

16

COMPOUND HETEROZYGOUS C677T & A1298C LABS

Remember, this is where they have one of each gene transcription error and moderate symptoms. The Spectracell™ testing we use looks at intracellular vitamins and minerals.

Patient 1

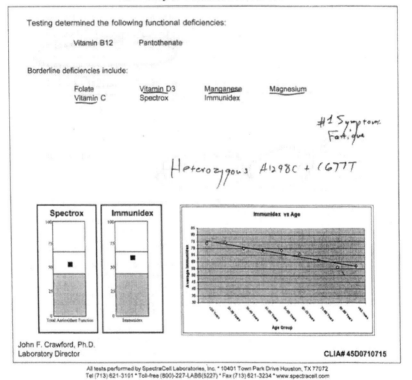

Intracellular

SpectraCell Laboratories
Science • Health • Solutions

LABORATORY REPORT

Account Number: 206649	Name:
	Gender: DOB: 02/07/1994
Danny Purser , M.D.	
383 W. 600 North	Accession Number:
Lindon, UT 84042	Requisition Number:
USA	
	Date of Collection: 05/21/2015
	Date Received: 05/22/2015
	Date Reported: 06/02/2015

Summary of Deficient Test Results

Testing determined the following functional deficiencies:

Vitamin B12   Pantothenate

Borderline deficiencies include:

Folate	Vitamin D3	Manganese	Magnesium
Vitamin C	Spectrox	Immunidex	

#1 Symptom:
Fatigue

Heterozygous A1298C + C677T

Spectrox	Immunidex	Immunidex vs Age

John F. Crawford, Ph.D.
Laboratory Director

CLIA# 45D0710715

All tests performed by SpectraCell Laboratories, Inc. * 10401 Town Park Drive Houston, TX 77072
Tel (713) 621-3101 * Toll-free (800)-227-LABS(5227) * Fax (713) 621-3234 * www.spectracell.com

Micronutrients	Patient Results (% Control)	Functional Abnormals	Reference Range (greater than)
B Complex Vitamins			
Vitamin B1 (Thiamin)	94		>78%
Vitamin B2 (Riboflavin)	69		>53%
Vitamin B3 (Niacinamide)	92		>80%
Vitamin B6 (Pyridoxine)	63		>54%
Vitamin B12 (Cobalamin)	14	Deficient	>14%
Folate	35	Borderline	>32%
Pantothenate	7	Deficient	>7%
Biotin	44		>34%
Amino Acids			
Serine	42		>30%
Glutamine	51		>37%
Asparagine	55		>39%
Metabolites			
Choline	27		>20%
Inositol	71		>58%
Carnitine	58		>48%
Fatty Acids			
Oleic Acid	77		>65%
Other Vitamins			
Vitamin D3 (Cholecalciferol)	52	Borderline	>50%
Vitamin A (Retinol)	78		>70%
Vitamin K2	40		>30%
Minerals			
Calcium	51		>38%
Manganese	53	Borderline	>50%
Zinc	45		>37%
Copper	52		>42%
Magnesium	42	Borderline	>37%
Carbohydrate Metabolism			
Glucose-Insulin Interaction	50		>38%
Fructose Sensitivity	43		>34%
Chromium	46		>40%
Antioxidants			
Glutathione	55		>42%
Cysteine	51		>41%
Coenzyme Q-10	93		>86%
Selenium	80		>74%
Vitamin E (A-tocopherol)	91		>84%
Alpha Lipoic Acid	89		>81%
Vitamin C	47	Borderline	>40%
SPECTROX™			
Total Antioxidant Function	54	Borderline	>40%
Proliferation Index			
Immunidex	58	Borderline	>40%

The reference ranges listed in the above table are valid for male and female patients 12 years of age or older.

SpectraCell Laboratories
Science • Health • Solutions
10401 Town Park Drive
Houston, TX 77072

Phone:	(713)621-3101
TollFree:	(800)227-LABS(5227)
Fax:	(281)568-5246

Laboratory Report

Account Number:	206649	Name:	▮▮▮▮▮		
		Gender:	M	DOB:	2/7/1994

Danny Purser , M.D.
383 W. 600 North

Lindon, UT 84042

Accession Number:	N85582
Requisition Number:	
Date Collected:	May 21, 2015
Date Received:	May 22, 2015
Date Reported:	June 3, 2015

MTHFR Genotype Test Result

Test	Result
C677T Mutation	Heterozygous
A1298C Mutation	Heterozygous

This sample has one copy of the C677T mutation and one copy of the A1298C mutation.
This genotype
 • is associated with decreased enzyme activity (approximately 50-60% of normal activity).
 • is associated with increased homocysteine levels.
 • is correlated with increased risk of cardiovascular disease or thrombosis.
 • is associated with potential methotrexate intolerance and patients may require dosage adjustments or
   discontinuation.

John F. Crawford, Ph.D.
Laboratory Director

CLIA# 45D0710715

MTHFR Background Information

MTHFR (methylenetetrahydrofolate reductase) is an enzyme involved in the metabolism of folate and homocysteine. It plays a role in maintaining cellular folate levels and is a cofactor needed to convert homocysteine (a potentially toxic amino acid) to methionine.
Certain common genetic point mutations have been characterized that reduce the function of the MTHFR enzyme. These are the C677T mutation (which is a change from cytosine to thymine at position 677 within the gene) and the A1298C mutation (which is a change from adenine to cytosine at position 1298 within the gene.) An MTHFR enzyme with reduced function can lead to elevated homocysteine levels, which is a known independent risk factor for development of cardiovascular disease and venous thrombosis. Reduced enzyme function can also affect folate status.
An additional area in which the function of MTHFR can have an effect is during methotrexate therapy. Methotrexate is a drug often used in treatment of certain cancers or autoimmune diseases. It is a structural analogue of folate and can interfere with folate metabolism. Defects in folate metabolism such as those potentially arising from mutations affecting MTHFR function can increase sensitivity to methotrexate and may lead to lower dosage requirements, increased side effects, or intolerance of the drug.

Testing Limitations

Only the C667T and A1298C mutations are analyzed in this assay. There may be other unknown non-genetic factors or genetic factors besides the tested mutations that can affect homocysteine levels, folate status, or drug sensitivities. Rare mutations in the primer binding sites used to detect the C677T and A1298C mutations may prevent detection. Specific dosing guidelines for methotrexate based on MTHFR genotype are not currently available.
MTHFR genotyping can provide useful information concerning risks of developing cardiovascular disease or thrombosis, or potential for increased sensitivity to methotrexate treatment. However, genotyping alone is not predictive of development of disease or complication and should not be used as the primary means of clinical diagnosis or treatment decision making. This information should be used by a physician in conjunction with additional clinical information to determine an appropriate treatment regimen.

SpectraCell Laboratories
Science • Health • Solutions

Patient 2

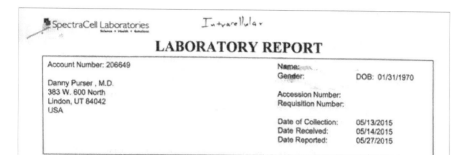

SpectraCell Laboratories *Intracellular*

LABORATORY REPORT

Account Number: 206649

Danny Purser , M.D.
383 W. 600 North
Lindon, UT 84042
USA

Name:
Gender: DOB: 01/31/1970

Accession Number:
Requisition Number:

Date of Collection: 05/13/2015
Date Received: 05/14/2015
Date Reported: 05/27/2015

Summary of Deficient Test Results

Testing determined the following functional deficiencies:

Biotin   Vitamin D3   Vitamin C

Borderline deficiencies include:

Vitamin B3	Vitamin B6	Vitamin B12	Folate
Pantothenate	Serine	Glutamine	Inositol
Carnitine	Fructose	Chromium	Cysteine
Vitamin K2	Spectrox	immunidex	

#1 Symptom: Fatigue

Heterozygous 1298c + C677T

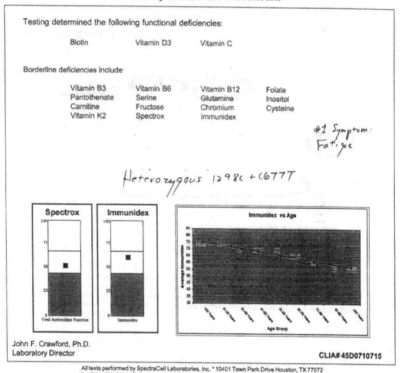

Spectrox   Immunidex   Immunidex vs Age

John F. Crawford, Ph.D.
Laboratory Director

CLIA# 45D0710715

All tests performed by SpectraCell Laboratories, Inc. * 10401 Town Park Drive Houston, TX 77072
Tel (713) 621-3101 * Toll-free (800)-227-LABS(5227) * Fax (713) 621-3234 * www.spectracell.com

SpectraCell Laboratories, Inc.
Laboratory Test Report   Accession Number:

Micronutrients	Patient Results (% Control)	Functional Abnormals	Reference Range (greater than)
B Complex Vitamins			
Vitamin B1 (Thiamin)	85		>78%
Vitamin B2 (Riboflavin)	71		>53%
Vitamin B3 (Niacinamide)	82	Borderline	>80%
Vitamin B6 (Pyridoxine)	58	Borderline	>54%
Vitamin B12 (Cobalamin)	17	Borderline	>14%
Folate	34	Borderline	>32%
Pantothenate	10	Borderline	>7%
Biotin	33	Deficient	>34%
Amino Acids			
Serine	33	Borderline	>30%
Glutamine	42	Borderline	>37%
Asparagine	54		>39%
Metabolites			
Choline	27		>20%
Inositol	62	Borderline	>58%
Carnitine	49	Borderline	>46%
Fatty Acids			
Oleic Acid	74		>65%
Other Vitamins			
Vitamin D3 (Cholecalciferol)	50	Deficient	>50%
Vitamin A (Retinol)	80		>70%
Vitamin K2	33	Borderline	>30%
Minerals			
Calcium	51		>38%
Manganese	64		>50%
Zinc	52		>37%
Copper	56		>42%
Magnesium	54		>37%
Carbohydrate Metabolism			
Glucose-Insulin Interaction	56		>38%
Fructose Sensitivity	36	Borderline	>34%
Chromium	44	Borderline	>40%
Antioxidants			
Glutathione	50		>42%
Cysteine	43	Borderline	>41%
Coenzyme Q-10	90		>86%
Selenium	79		>74%
Vitamin E (A-tocopherol)	89		>84%
Alpha Lipoic Acid	87		>81%
Vitamin C	37	Deficient	>40%
SPECTROX™			
Total Antioxidant Function	52	Borderline	>40%
Proliferation Index			
Immunidex	58	Borderline	>40%

The reference ranges listed in the above table are valid for male and female patients 12 years of age or older.

SpectraCell Laboratories
Science • Health • Solutions
10401 Town Park Drive
Houston, TX 77072

Phone:	(713)621-3101
TollFree:	(800)227-LABS(5227)
Fax:	(281)568-5246

Laboratory Report

Account Number:	206649	Name:		
		Gender:	DOB:	1/31/1970

Danny Purser , M.D.
383 W. 600 North

Lindon, UT 84042

Accession Number:
Requisition Number:

Date Collected:	May 13, 2015
Date Received:	May 14, 2015
Date Reported:	May 18, 2015

MTHFR Genotype Test Result

Test	Result
C677T Mutation	Heterozygous
A1298C Mutation	Heterozygous

This sample has one copy of the C677T mutation and one copy of the A1298C mutation.
This genotype

- is associated with decreased enzyme activity (approximately 50-60% of normal activity).
- is associated with increased homocysteine levels.
- is correlated with increased risk of cardiovascular disease or thrombosis.
- is associated with potential methotrexate intolerance and patients may require dosage adjustments or discontinuation.

John F. Crawford, Ph.D.
Laboratory Director

CLIA# 45D0710715

MTHFR Background Information

MTHFR (methylenetetrahydrofolate reductase) is an enzyme involved in the metabolism of folate and homocysteine. It plays a role in maintaining cellular folate levels and is a cofactor needed to convert homocysteine (a potentially toxic amino acid) to methionine.

Certain common genetic point mutations have been characterized that reduce the function of the MTHFR enzyme. These are the C677T mutation (which is a change from cytosine to thymine at position 677 within the gene) and the A1298C mutation (which is a change from adenine to cytosine at position 1298 within the gene.) An MTHFR enzyme with reduced function can lead to elevated homocysteine levels, which is a known independent risk factor for development of cardiovascular disease and venous thrombosis. Reduced enzyme function can also affect folate status.

An additional area in which the function of MTHFR can have an effect is during methotrexate therapy. Methotrexate is a drug often used in treatment of certain cancers or autoimmune diseases. It is a structural analogue of folate and can interfere with folate metabolism. Defects in folate metabolism such as those potentially arising from mutations affecting MTHFR function can increase sensitivity to methotrexate and may lead to lower dosage requirements, increased side effects, or intolerance of the drug.

Testing Limitations

Only the C667T and A1298C mutations are analyzed in this assay. There may be other unknown non-genetic factors or genetic factors besides the tested mutations that can affect homocysteine levels, folate status, or drug sensitivities. Rare mutations in the primer binding sites used to detect the C677T and A1298C mutations may prevent detection. Specific dosing guidelines for methotrexate based on MTHFR genotype are not currently available.

MTHFR genotyping can provide useful information concerning risks of developing cardiovascular disease or thrombosis, or potential for increased sensitivity to methotrexate treatment. However, genotyping alone is not predictive of development of disease or complication and should not be used as the primary means of clinical diagnosis or treatment decision making. This information should be used by a physician in conjunction with additional clinical information to determine an appropriate treatment regimen.

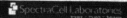

Visit us at www.spectracell.com or call us at 800.227.LABS (5227)

SpectraCell Laboratories

Treatment is the same as if they have Homozygus C677T. But my experience is they may have slightly fewer issues, and sometimes you cannot go up as high or as fast on the main "methylation support". But regardless, treat them like Homzygous   C677T.

17

OTHER GENETIC PROBLEMS?

YOU MAY NOTICE you have positive markers for something called COMT on your 23andme® DNA results.

COMT H62H rs4633 RESULTS: ++

COMT V158M rs4680 RESULTs: ++

MAO A R297R rs6323 TYPICAL RESULTS: +

First, people with MAO and COMT are predisposed to simply have TOO MUCH ADRENALINE in the body. They tend to overreact to stressors, plus have more pain to stimuli.

COMT MAIN PROBLEM: Being homozygous for COMT gives a 700% (seven fold) increased risk for breast cancer. Please look at treatment options for these women at the end of this chapter, as there are ways to offset this.

MAO-A MAIN PROBLEM: This is called the "Warrior Gene" because it is felt to cause increased aggression in men and women with this gene. Monoamine Oxidase A is an enzyme that in humans is encoded by the MAOA gene.[57] [58] This gene is one of two neighboring gene family members that encode mitochondrial enzymes which catalyze the oxidative deamination of amines, such as dopamine, norepinephrine, and serotonin. Mutation of this gene results in Brunner syndrome.[59] This gene has also been associated with a variety of other psychiatric disorders, including antisocial behavior.

Other Major Problems Related to COMT and MAO

This excellent review is from Dr. Andrew Rostenberg, D.C. at Red Mountain Natural Medicine Clinic[60] in Boise, Idaho, and is very appropriate, though I've added an addition or two below. His treatment protocol is also very helpful (see below also).

"Anything that powerful must be kept under tight control, otherwise we will develop other issues that can damage our health. Some common issues that result from too much adrenaline:

Insomnia – people with too little catecholamines are narcoleptic, they can fall asleep anywhere; those with too many catecholamines simply can't turn their mind off and lay awake for hours!

Chronic Pain – pain fibers become more sensitive in the presence of adrenaline, leading to syndromes like fibromyalgia and allodynia; this may cause pain just walking around the block, doing the dishes or rolling over in bed.

High Blood Pressure – adrenaline increases the rate and force of the heart; excess adrenaline will raise blood pressure – think bulging veins on side of forehead when someone is filled with rage!

POTS and other sympathetic disorders – while the causes of these issue may be complex, they each involve imbalances of the catecholamine stress hormones.

Arrhythmia – excess stress placed on the heart often depletes the heart of taurine, magnesium, and nitric oxide; this causes an epilepsy-like effect on heart; that is arrhythmia should be considered a seizure of the heart.

Excess Sweating – adrenaline activates skin receptors to cause sweating

Tingling and Numbness – excess catecholamines (adrenaline) can cause tingling and numbness on both sides of the body, in the hands and feet; this may mimic neuropathy, but is just a side effect of excess adrenaline on the nervous system.

Poor Circulation – adrenaline pushes blood away from the gut and can cut off flow to the tips of our fingers; for example people with Raynaud's phenomenon have so much adrenaline that it shuts off the flow of blood completely, leaving the skin white and cold.

Digestion Problems – since adrenaline pushes blood away from the gut, people with MAO and COMT may suffer from IBS; for with less blood there is less oxygen, and we cannot properly digest our food. Bacteria in the gut also use adrenaline to grow very rapidly.

OCD, Anger, Mood Changes and Anxiety – the increase of adrenaline comes at the expense of the loss of dopamine; every molecule of adrenaline is first a molecule of dopamine and so whenever the body produces excess adrenaline/noradrenaline, it will lower the available dopamine. High adrenaline with low dopamine doesn't feel good, and may make you cranky and hard to be around.

Low Thyroid – tyrosine is used to make dopamine, and dopamine is used to make adrenaline; tyrosine is also used to make thyroid hormone, so when we are stressed, thyroid function often drops as there is less tyrosine available to make T3 and T4."[61]

Increased Breast Cancer – several studies have shown that COMT variants especially the val108met variant of COMT, are associated with a 3-4 times increased risk for breast cancer – that's VERY significant. Properly increasing your folate levels seems to offset this risk.

How to Treat or Deal With COMT and MAO?

Four Ways to Manage Your MAO and COMT Genes (by Dr. Andrew Rostenberg, D.C.):

1) Calm down gut inflammation by avoiding food allergens and processed, garbage GMO foods. Shop the outside of the supermarket, avoiding the isles. There is no one perfect diet for everyone but as Michael Pollen said, "eat food, mostly plants, not too much." You may need to consider digestive aids and anti-inflammatory supplements and foods to help reduce inflammation even more. 70% of inflammation comes from the gut, so taking care of digestion is always the first priority.

2) Exercise moderately as this creates a calming, relaxation response in the nervous system. However, one must avoid working out after 7pm as it raises adrenaline. People with MAO and COMT are going to have a difficult time sleeping after a workout that ends at 8 or 9 pm. We can do that when we are 10 years old, but the older we get, the more sensitive we become.

3) Get 8-9 hours of sleep. Most people need 7 hours minimum. Often people who are recovering from an acute or chronic illness need more like 8-9 hours of sleep to optimize their healing and wellness.

4) Avoid unnecessary stress and take time for yourself. Learn to say no to stressful situations. Recharging your batteries is not selfish; rather it allows you to be your best which helps you help others. If we are sick and tired, how much of an asset can we be to someone else?

Because the side effects of too much stress are so damaging, people with MAO and COMT must be very careful to manage stress effectively. "[62]

Another option is to add magnesium and to make sure your Spectracell® Micronutrient Panel does not show any copper or manganese deficiencies and if so, to deal with those. Small doses of Magnesium Glycinate (200 mg to 400 mg) can also help, sometimes alot.[63] (Watch for low BP.)

MY TREATMENT OF COMT and MAO-A:

It's simple – a number of studies and experts have concluded that natural progesterone usage really calms these people down and is the treatment of choice.[64] If serum levels in women are maintained above 20 ng/dl reduces breast cancer risk of death by 500%.[65]

It should be used with these people if they desire, mostly to help sleep or as a natural anxiolytic. It is widely available through better compounding pharmacies – the best in the world is MedQuest in Bountiful, Utah (http://www.mqrx.com). MedQuest also offers courses (based on the peer reviewed literature) taught by the entertaining and very popular Dr. Neal Rouzier on hormone usage and prescribing that receive rave reviews.

I've also had my biggest #1 book ever (it still sells many copies) on this very subject – called **PROGESTERONE: THE WOMEN'S ULTIMATE FEEL GOOD HORMONE** (by Dan Purser MD).

I've also had two very popular online educational courses on progesterone research, usage, pharmacology and prescribing for the public and doctors too. One course was for Natural **Progesterone Therapy For PMS, Endometriosis, and Menstrual Migraines** and the other was for **Natural Progesterone Usage In Menopause**.

Here are the URLs if you wish to take one:

http://drpursercourse.com/evergreen-page0-start

http://drpursercourse.com/prog-mini-buy-now

Problem solved.

?

18

WHERE DOES PYRIDOXINE (B6) FIT?

Hard to get better than this summary by Donna Johnson, RN at MTHFR Alliance – please check it out.

"Have MTHFR, CBS, BHMT and/or SHMT mutations?

Folate and B12 or other supplements not helping? You may just need more B6 than you previously thought.

There are 56 (56!) B6-Dependent Enzymes in the body. MTHFR, CBS, BHMT and SHMT are acronyms for some key enzymes, and those are 4 of 56 that depend on plenty of B6. Here's the rub: B6-Dependent enzymes are inhibited or paralyzed in a state of Oxidative Stress! What does that mean? Your B6 levels could be "normal" on your NutrEval® (for example) but because of Oxidative Stress, that "normal" level of B6 is made mostly unavailable to the enzymes that depend on it. *[AUTHOR NOTE: Not sure what a NutrEval® is but this is why I always get*

INTRACELLULAR testing via Spectracell™ Comprehensive Micronutrient Panel before starting anything.]

As important as having sufficient B6 on board is, it's critical to note that B6 and Magnesium work together on enzyme pathways – they are an Alliance! Typically, for every 1mg of B6, at least 2-3 mg of Magnesium is recommended. Now, back to why Folate, B12 or other Methylation supplements may not be doing anything for your Methylation/Detoxification Pathway. Methionine sits at the very beginning of this Methylation Cycle. And Methionine Synthase is one of the enzymes severely affected by insufficient B6 in a state of Oxidative Stress."

What else is B6 responsible for? Making serotonin, converting glutamate into calming GABA, making dopamine... any light-bulbs going off for anyone? We hope so! Here's a great summary of what other things B6 is responsible for:

http://lpi.oregonstate.edu/infocenter/
vitamins/vitaminB6/

*Just remember, this article does not take into account the role that Oxidative Stress plays on B6.

So, how do you know how much B6 your body needs? How do you know how much Oxidative Stress is making your B6 unavailable? There are over 100 markers on an Organic Acids Urine Test (Oat) and some of those markers, particularly glycolic acid, go up when there is insufficient B6.

But now we come to one of the greater tragedies in modern medicine. We in the medical field have long trusted laboratory values and testing methods to guide us. But all labs are still using an antiquated, completely unreliable marker – creatinine – to measure ALL of the other urinary markers against. This is a 100-year old theory, using the work of ONE scientist's theory on creatinine, and his theory about creatinine's reliability was proven wrong years ago! Creatinine is a highly unreliable marker to measure other markers against. (You may want to read that creatinine bit again. It takes a while to sink in.) So, if the labs aren't using the right thing(s) to measure everything else in your Oat, UAA, or other urine test markers against, how far reaching would the downstream problems and mistakes then be? Ponder it!

Now to the next potential glitch with B6. After B6 goes through digestion, it turns into P5P and back into B6 again via something called phosphorylation – which is just the adding and removing a phosphate group. This requires 2 different enzymes. Some of us may lack the enzyme that adds the phosphate group, so we may do well on P5P. Some of us may lack the other enzyme that takes the phosphate group off and might do better with B6.

Figuring out what form or forms are best for you, may take a little trial and error – unfortunately there's no way to know which form(s) are best suited for your body. We at MTHFR Alliance® are committed to helping you figure out just how severe your B6 and Magnesium insufficiency and/or deficiency is. These are some of the most critical, yet commonly overlooked, first steps on the road back to better health."[66]

So when and how do you take B6 (pyridoxine)?

In Chapter 19 we also discuss the Methylfolate Trap and overdose of methylfolate – which causes aches, pains, nausea, sharp (or even dull) headaches. This is when you should try reducing your methylfolate dose and adding B3 (niacin) or B6 (pyridoxine).

Remember a zinc deficiency makes taking B6 worthless. Go back and look at your most recent Spectracell™ Comprehensive Micronutrient Panel and if your zinc was low add Optizinc™ first please.

Next you can try taking B6 from 25-100 mg a day based on your original homocysteine level. This is an interesting diagram from MTHFR Living blog.[67]

Daily Nutrient Needs Based on Homocysteine Score

NUTRIENT HIGH RISK	NO RISK	LOW RISK	HIGH RISK	VERY HIGH RISK
Hcy Lvl 15	H<6	6-9	9-15	Above 15
Folate	200mcg	400mcg	1,200mcg	2,000mcg
B12	10mcg	500mcg	1,000mcg	1,500mcg
B6	25mg	50mg	75mg	100mg
B2	10mg	15mg	20mg	50mg
Zinc	5mg	10mg	20mg	20mg
Magnesium	100mg	200mg	300mg	400mg
TMG	500mg	750mg	1.5-3g	3-6g

What Do You Take if You Need B6?

I like Source Naturals™ Coenzymated B-6 Sublingual 25mg, 60 Count on Amazon™ – as natural as you can get. Try one to begin with, but may take as many as 4.

If I had MTHFR I'd have a bottle of B6 around just for emergencies.

⁂

19

THE METHYLFOLATE TRAP

A PHYSIOLOGICAL RESPONSE in man to prevent methyl group deficiency in kwashiorkor (methionine deficiency) and an explanation for folic-acid induced exacerbation of subacute combined degeneration in pernicious anemia.

Though not much discussed in MTHFR circles, pernicious anemia is a major side effect of chronic B12 deficiency (as in MTHFR disease).

Conversely if you have pernicious anemia then you might very well (and probably do) have MTHFR - a fact rarely if ever discussed, pondered or even considered by hematologists or medical doctors in general (yes, I am a western medical doctor and yes, I've missed this connection more than once in my earlier life – and I'm sorry for that, too).

From Medline Plus here's the definition of pernicious anemia (NOTE that MTHFR is not mentioned anywhere):

"PERNICIOUS ANEMIA"

Anemia is a condition in which the body does not have enough healthy red blood cells. Red blood cells provide oxygen to body tissues. There are many types of anemia.

Pernicious anemia is a decrease in red blood cells that occurs when the intestines cannot properly absorb vitamin B12.

Causes

Pernicious anemia is a type of vitamin B12 anemia. The body needs vitamin B12 to make red blood cells. You get this vitamin from eating foods such as meat, poultry, shellfish, eggs, and dairy products.

A special protein, called intrinsic factor (IF), helps your intestines absorb vitamin B12. This protein is released by cells in the stomach. When the stomach does not make enough intrinsic factor, the intestine cannot properly absorb vitamin B12.

Common causes of pernicious anemia include:

Weakened stomach lining (atrophic gastritis).

An autoimmune condition in which the body's immune system attacks the actual intrinsic factor protein or the cells in the lining of your stomach that make it.

Very rarely, pernicious anemia is passed down through families. This is called congenital pernicious anemia. Babies with this type of anemia do not make enough intrinsic factor. Or they cannot properly absorb vitamin B12 in the small intestine.

In adults, symptoms of pernicious anemia are usually not seen until after age 30. The average age of diagnosis is age 60.

You are more likely to get this disease if you:

> Are Scandinavian or Northern European
> Have a family history of the condition

Certain diseases can also raise your risk. They include:

> Addison disease
> Chronic thyroiditis
> Graves disease
> Hypoparathyroidism
> Hypopituitarism
> Myasthenia gravis
> Secondary amenorrhea
> Type 1 diabetes
> Testicular dysfunction
> Vitiligo[68]

Family History? Northern European? Endocrine problems? Sounds like the population of MTHFR patients. The hematologists should rethink this one.

Regardless, to prevent a Methylfolate Trap from occurring, a patient with MTHFR will decreases SAM to prevent this from occurring.

> "It is suggested that in man the methylfolate trap is a normal physiological response to impending methyl group deficiency resulting from a very low supply of methionine. This decreases cellular S-adenosyl-

methionine (SAM) [i.e. SAMe – author], which puts at risk important methylation reactions, including those required to maintain myelin. In order to protect these methylation reactions, the cell has evolved two mechanisms to maintain supplies of methionine and SAM as a first priority. (a) Decreased SAM causes the folate co-factors to be directed through the cycle involving 5-methyl-tetrahydrofolate (5-methyl-THF) and methionine synthetase and away from the cycles that produce purines and pyrimidines for DNA synthesis. This enhances the remethylation of homocysteine to methionine and SAM. In addition, by restricting DNA biosynthesis and with it cell division competition for methionine for protein synthesis is reduced. Thus, whatever methionine is available is conserved for the vital methylation reactions in the nerves, brain, and elsewhere. (b) 5-methyl-THF, the form in which almost all folate is transported in human plasma, must react with intracellular homocysteine before it can be retained by the cell as a polyglutamate. Since homocysteine is derived entirely from methionine, methionine deficiency will cause intracellular folate deficiency, and the rate of mitosis of rapidly dividing cells will be reduced. Although these two processes have evolved as a response to methionine deficiency, they also occur in B12 deficiency, which the cell mistakenly interprets as lack of methionine. The resulting response is inappropriate and gives rise to a potentially lethal anemia. In these circumstances the methylation reactions are also partly protected by the reduced rate of cell division.

This explains why administration of folic acid [NOTE: this is considered toxic to to MTHFR patients - author], which induces cell division and use of methionine in protein synthesis, impairs methylation of myelin and precipitates or exacerbates subacute combined degeneration (SCD). During folate deficiency methionine biosynthesis is also diminished. As in methionine deficiency, the body responds to decreasing availability of SAM by diverting folate away from DNA biosynthesis towards the remethylation of homocysteine to methionine and SAM. The selective use of available folate to conserve methionine, together with the ability of nerve tissue to concentrate folate form the plasma, explains the absence of SCD in folate deficiency."[69]

Symptoms

The symptoms of this, in my experience are fatigue, sharp headaches, muscle aches and pains, and nausea.

If this occurs, this is because you are probably taking TOO much methylfolate too soon.

Hold, then reduce your methylfolate dramatically and try small doses of niacin 50 mg – the B3 can get rid of the trap and help with the methylfolate overdose.

Drink lots of fluids, adding some green tea.

Dr. Ben Lynch at MTHFR.net advises the same.

"Side Effects and Toxicity of Methylfolate: In doses typically administered for therapeutic purposes, 5-MTHF is considered non-toxic. At doses of up to 50 mg daily, gastrointestinal complaints, insomnia, irritability, and fatigue have been mentioned as occasional side effects. Folic acid and 5-MTHF are considered safe during pregnancy, with a recommended intake of 800 mcg daily.

To answer your questions:

1) The metafolin is going to be directly absorbed just like the methylfolate – sublingually.

2) Taking too much of anything is not good. Is taking too much methylfolate dangerous? In most people, no. It is not going to cause long term issues or death or a serious health concern – and not even any side effects.

People take upwards of 50 mg of methylfolate daily for their depression or other mental dysfunctions.

I am very conservative when it comes to dose suggestions as I don't like people being 'macho' and thinking that if they take 10 mg of methylfolate, that will be better than 1 mg. Sometimes yes it will and sometimes it won't.

What could you experience if you do take too much methylfolate?

- ➤ Irritability
- ➤ Anxiety
- ➤ Nausea
- ➤ Headaches
- ➤ Insomnia

Will these symptoms go away upon reducing the levels of methylfolate or stopping it?

Yes

Will these symptoms go away quickly?

In most people – yes – these symptoms will stop within 24 hours if not earlier.

Can you 'neutralize' these side effects faster if they occur?

Many times, yes.

How?

➤ By taking niacin, as niacin binds methyl groups and also increases the breakdown of glutamate – which is the excitatory neurotransmitter.

➤ By taking vitamin B6 – for many people – as B6 converts glutamate to GABA and GABA is the inhibitory neurotransmitter.

You can see how GABA can help with depression, anxiety, and calming:

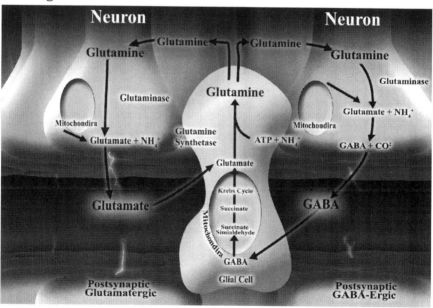

As a physician, it is my job to:

> ➤ Do no harm
> ➤ Inform
> ➤ Educate

That said – I encourage people to start low and work up carefully to avoid these side effects.

If I have 'scared' you – in a way, that is good – because you – and others – will take my recommendations to go slowly seriously."[70]

An interesting YouTube Video on this subject:

https://www.youtube.com/watch?v=cU1U7nkUPv8

20

A1298C HOMOZYGOUS MUTATION THERAPY

LESS COMMON THAN a C677T (and far worse in many ways) is the A1298C MTHFR Homozygous mutation (meaning you have TWO A1298C mutations or SNPS).

This Homozygous variant only causes a decline of about 30% in the methylation (versus a 60-70% decline in the C7677T Homozygous variant and 40% decline with the Heterozygous variant) but comes with its own set of unique problems beyond all that, and they're much more psychological but no less troublesome.

Symptoms exist, and there is definitely a correlation when there are confirmed MTHFR A1298C Homozygous errors. But even if you are Heterozygous (have both the A1298C and the C677T), the A1298C SNP can still cause symptoms to bleed through.

So, as I said, (and Dr. Ben Lynch of MTHFR.net agrees), the MTHFR A1298C mutation may affect you if you are either:

> Homozygous A1298C MTHFR mutation
> Compound Heterozygous A1298C + C677T MTHFR mutation

I know many doctors evaluate homocysteine only when it comes to MTHFR mutations – you hopefully see now how that's a mistake – especially in this case.

Those with A1298C MTHFR mutations do not display elevated homocysteine unless they are combined with C677T. Even when combined with C677T MTHFR mutations, the A1298C types still do not tend to have very elevated homocysteine levels.

PROBLEMS FROM A1298C HOMOZYGOUS

Mood Disorders

Mood disorders in MTHFR are not confined to people with A1298C MTHFR, just as Homocysteine elevations are not confined just to C677T Homozygous mutations.

But if your BH4 cycle is not working properly due to a MTHFR mutation, you are definitely going to be expressing some symptoms either mentally, emotionally or physically – or – all together.

SYMPTOMS often associated with A1298C MTHFR mutations:

> Hypertension
> Delayed Speech
> Muscle Pain
> Insomnia
> Irritable Bowel Syndrome

- Fibromyalgia
- Chronic Fatigue Syndrome
- Hand Tremor
- Memory Loss
- Headaches
- Brain Fog

SIGNS often associated with A1298C MTHFR Mutations:

- Elevated Ammonia Levels
- Decreased Dopamine
- Decreased Serotonin
- Decreased Epinephrine And Norepinephrine
- Decreased Nitric Oxide
- Elevated Blood Pressure
- Muscle Tenderness
- Ulcers
- Pre-Eclampsia (During Pregnancy)

CONDITIONS associated with A1298C MTHFR mutations:

- Fibromyalgia
- Chronic Fatigue Syndrome
- Autism
- Depression
- Insomnia
- ADD/ADHD
- Irritable Bowel Syndrome

➤ Inflammatory Bowel Syndrome
➤ Erectile Dysfunction
➤ Migraine
➤ Raynaud's
➤ Cancer
➤ Alzheimer's
➤ Parkinson's
➤ Recurrent Miscarriages

NOTE:

That The BH4 cycle is absolutely critical
for these various functions:

---

1.   Assists the breakdown of phenylalanine
2.   Helps form these neurotransmitters:
    i.   Serotonin
    ii.   Melatonin
    iii. Dopamine
    iv. Norepinephrine (noradrenaline)
    v.   Epinephrine (adrenaline)
        Cofactor to produce Nitric Oxide (NO)
        Manufacture of CoQ10.

Regardless of which snp you have, either the 677 or 1298, the MTHFR enzyme's end product, methylfolate, supports two major pathways: BH4 and Methylation.

What is BH4?[71]

BH4 – Tetrahydrobiopterin (also called biopterin or tetrabiopterin)

The Basics

BH4 is an enzyme that is used to make serotonin, dopamine, thyroid hormones, melanin (patients tend to be pale) and to detox ammonia (thus a decline in BH4 could cause mental or psychological disorders). BH4 is recharged by folate and/or niacin and/or vitamin C. With certain combinations of the MTHFR gene involving A1298C, some people have a limited supply of BH4. *Those people can probably be identified as those who have tendencies towards depression, low energy, all-or-nothing focus, hypothyroid (even subclinical), are pale, and may have elevated blood ammonia.* (Clinicians need to watch for these individuals.)

IMPORTANT: These people will do best on small amounts of very high quality protein, and lots of methyl folate or more importantly – FOLINIC ACID (read below). SO TRY FOLINIC ACID FIRST AND FOREMOST.

Reasons to Suspect Low BH4

Suspect it if you have low dopamine AND low serotonin AND low thyroid function (i.e. hypothyroidism or even subclinical hypothyroidism), or if you have high blood ammonia, or if you have MTHFR polymorphisms, especially ones that involve A1298C.

Sources of BH4

Vitamins/Supplements That Help:

The main way to increase BH4 is by recycling it from Folate (or the more natural Folinic Acid – read below), Niacin, Methylfolate (i.e. Folinic Acid in this case), SAMe, and/or Vitamin C.

THINGS TO CONSIDER WITH HOMOZYGOUS A1298C PATIENTS:

➤ Start with methionine 500 mgm capsules first. If two each day are well tolerated then change to SAMe (and avoid extra methylfolate or especially folic acid!) at one to two per day.

➤ Niacin should be supplemented at 50 mg a day in multiple doses – again on Amazon™ – from Seeking Health™ at 50 mg for Nicotinic Acid 100 vegetable caps.

➤ Folinic acid is available on Amazon™ (I'll talk more about it later in this chapter) - MegaFolinic™, 800 Mcg 120 Tablets from Source Naturals™. Start with one but go up from there.

➤ I have actually seen several cases of scurvy here in the USA (I know, surprising but true) so in addition to everything else please try this version of Vitamin C on Amazon™ - Nutrigold™ Vitamin C Gold™ (Made from Non-GMO, Organic Berries and Fruits - NOT Synthetic Ascorbic Acid), 240 mg, 90 veg capsules — I think this is the BEST Vitamin C on the market!

➤ 5-HTP at night, before bed, can raise BH4 levels (and help sleep) – there are dozens of studies that show this in severe infantile cases[72] but it is unclear whether it has lasting benefits in adults with milder forms of BH4 deficiency. I prefer this brand and smaller dose version (50 mg) made by Source Naturals™ - Source Naturals™ 5-HTP, 50mg, 60 Capsules.

➤ Light Therapy can also affect and improve the production of BH4 and help with SAD (Seasonal Affective Disorder). (Tetrahydrobiopterin or BH4 is an essential cofactor in the hydroxylation of tryptophan and therefore in the synthesis of serotonin, while neopterin is known as a marker of cell-mediated immune activity.)[73] I and my patients like this light the best on Amazon™ - Lightphoria™ 10,000LUX Energy Light Lamp from Sphere Gadget Technologies (look at the reviews – wow!).

➤ You may have to add Coq10 – I prefer ubiquinol because it's absorbed better than ubiquinone. My preferred Coq10 is Qunol™. Take two per day.

What is GTP?

"Guanosine-5'-triphosphate (GTP) is a purine nucleoside triphosphate. It can act as a substrate for the synthesis of RNA during the transcription process or DNA during DNA replication. Its structure is similar to that of the guanine nucleobase, the only difference being that nucleotides like GTP have a ribose sugar and three phosphates, with the nucleobase attached to the 1' and the triphosphate moiety attached to the 5' carbons of the ribose.

It also has the role of a source of energy or an activator of substrates in metabolic reactions, like that of ATP, but more specific. It is used as a source of energy for protein synthesis and gluconeogenesis.

GTP is involved in energy transfer within the cell. For instance, a GTP molecule is generated by one of the enzymes in the citric acid cycle. This is tantamount to the generation of one molecule of ATP, since GTP is readily converted to ATP with nucleoside-diphosphate kinase (NDK)."[74]

However, Too Much Protein In Diet Depletes BH4

Also, the body makes ammonia when it processes protein, and the BH4 pool is depleted when it detoxes that ammonia. Limiting dietary protein to the RDA (recommended daily amount) is the most effective way to keep ammonia levels reasonable.

To calculate the RDA go to this website to input your specific numbers into their calculator:

http://www.globalrph.com/protein-calculator.htm

For example, using the above calculator:

TYPICAL MALE PROTEIN RDA

- ➢ 40 years old
- ➢ 200 pounds
- ➢ Involved in some exercise

50% (if healthy) could survive on a minimum of 60 grams of protein/day

97-98% (if healthy) could survive on a minimum of 72.7 grams of protein/day

So, IF you're a MALE with Homozygous A1298C you'd want to keep at 60-73 grams of protein per day (say under 75 grams per day to make it easy).

TYPICAL FEMALE PROTEIN RDA

- ➢ 40 years old
- ➢ 150 pounds
- ➢ Involved in some exercise

50% (if healthy) could survive on a minimum of 45 grams of protein/day

97-98% (if healthy) could survive on a minimum of 54.6 grams of protein/day

So, IF you're a FEMALE with Homozygous A1298C you'd want to keep at 45-55 grams of protein per day (say under 60 grams per day to make it easy).

Does This Just Occur In A1298C Homozygous?

Most health care professionals think (who know about this even remotely – not many) that difficulty with BH4 regeneration/formation is only suffered by those having the

MTHFR A1298C snp – and not those with the MTHFR C677T snps.

This is incorrect.

Tetrahydrobiopterin (BH4) recycling is not just limited to those with A1298C compared to those with C677T.

In fact, lower BH4 levels are found more frequently in those with the C677T variant compared to the A1298C.

Why? Because the MTHFR 677 homozygous variant is more severe than the 1298.[75]

Lead and Aluminum

Formation of BH4 is impeded and reduced by LEAD and ALUMINUM.

5-formylTHF (Folinic Acid) is definitely needed in addition to 5-methylTHF (MethylFolate or 5-MTHF) or instead of.

What Is Folinic Acid? The Body's Folate

FOLINIC ACID: also known as 5-formyl tetrahydrofolate, is one active form in a group of vitamins known as folates. In contrast to folic acid, a synthetic form of folate, folinic acid is one of the forms of folate found naturally in foods. In the body folinic acid may be converted into any of the other active forms of folate.

Compared to folic acid, folinic acid is expensive, costing about 100 times more. However, the fact that the body only requires small amounts (less than one mg) means that one can obtain a two month supply of folinic acid for less than $10.

Folinic acid (mixed with 5-MTHF) is available on Amazon™ - MegaFolinic™, 800 Mcg 120 Tablets from Source Naturals™ but you'd need maybe at most one per day if you have A1298C.

Folinic acid has been available as a supplement for more than 10 years and as such has been the form most used as a replacement for folic acid.

5-MTHF: also known as L-5-methyl tetrahydrofolate has been difficult to obtain until recently. An Italian company has made a patented form available (Quatrefolic®) that is combined with a vegetarian glucosamine. This form is particularly stable and highly bioavailable. It is also in most of the supplements I have suggested throughout this book.

5-MTHF costs about 400 times more than folic acid. However, because the body requires less than one milligram (1 mg) on a daily basis, a person can buy a two-month supply for about $20.

5-MTHF is now readily available on the market, thereby making it possible to purchase at reasonable prices both coenzyme forms of folate.[76] I have taken advantage of this and use folinic acid (which includes both 5-MTHF and folinic acid).

Dr. Jill Carnahan feels that MTHFR suffferers do better on the natural version of folate – folinic acid:

"Some MTHFR cases prefer and do much better on the more natural folinic acid. And actually many patients like taking both – L-5-MTHF AND folinic acid but both must be given in really small doses just to begin with and for the duration of treatment[77] (forever?)."[78] [Dr. Carnahan's site is awesome and well worth the read.]

Can You Take BH4 (Biopterin or Tetrahydrobiopterin)?

Yes, for this situation (A1298C) the ideal dose is 2.5 mg up to four times per day. ("The effective dose of BH4 varies from 1 to 2 mg per kg-1 daily in patients with defective biopterin synthesis, to 5 mg per kg-1 or more in patients with dihydropteridine reductase (DHPR) deficiency. The cost of 2 mg per kg-1 day-1 of BH4 is comparable to the cost of a low Phenylalanine diet.")[79]

But BH4 is very hard to find, and when you do it is quite expensive.

If money is not an issue, here are the only two sources I know of for it:

Pteridin-4[80] at $79.50 for 60 capsules of 2.5mg BH4 – so a month's worth (4/day) would be two bottles or 120 capsules.

There is also a supplement available on Amazon® that contains a small amount (only 25 mcg) of BH4 (Biopterin) along with an appropriate addition of N-Acetyl-Tyrosine – it's called Ecological Formulas - Norival® (by Cardiovascular Research, LTD).

BH4 Labs?

You can easily test this level with Metametrix™ Neopterin/Biopterin Urine test – it's easy and not too expensive.

Or you can get the same test through Genova™ (you can easily find a doctor who offers Genova™ in your area).

OTHER Labs?

If you're in this boat or want to dig deeper – consider getting the Genova™ ION Profile with 40 Amino Acids testing performed. It's very helpful.

PROTOCOL FOR HOMOZYGOUS A1298C

It is hard to make a stepwise approach to this, so please understand this is just a rough attempt at this that I hope some of you will find helpful. I also cannot factor in everyone's finances so I'm assuming everyone has the money to do all of this – I am sorry if you don't - truly.

1. Signs? Symptoms? Conditions? Do these all match MTHFR especially the Homozygous A1298C variant?

2. Get a Spectracell™ Comprehensive Micronutrient Panel – this is INTRACELLULAR, so it is incredibly accurate - get this from a doctor who is signed up as a Spectracell™ provider. Carefully treat the deficiencies (see examples in this chapter) with the proper vitamins and supplements for your condition.

3. Also add a Homocysteine Level, and Whole Blood Histamine Level (to determine methylation capabilities).

4. Get a Metametrix™ or Genova™ Biopterin/Neopterin Urine panel – very helpful to se where you're at in the spectrum.

5. Get a Genova™ ION™ Profile with 40 Amino Acids – it helps to detail what else might be going on. This could come in very handy later.

6. Obtain and perform a salivary http://23andme.com genetic profile on yourself so you know what other mutations and enzymes you just might have.

7. Assuming you're Homozygous for A1298C, tighten your diet with the amount of protein you ingest.

8. Add moderately high purine foods to your diet too; such as Asparagus, Bacon, Beef, Cauliflower, Chicken, Chicken soup, Crab, Ham, Kidney beans, Lamb, Lentils, Lima beans, Lobster, Mushrooms, Mutton, Navy beans, Oatmeal, Peas, Pork, Salmon, Sheep, Spinach, Trout, Tuna, and Turkey.

9. Add broad spectrum light therapy daily for 15-20 minutes – start low and build-up slowly. In the depths of winter go longer if need be.

10. (REMEMBER - if whole blood histamine is LOW, the individual will be overmethylated. And if it is HIGH, they will be undermethylated.)

11. ★(FOR KIDS WITH ASD) Undermethylator (High Whole Blood Histamine Level >70 ng/ml) – SAMe works for these! It really does make them happy (but start on methionine trial

first 200-500 mg). DO NOT give your kids folate/folic acid! Also antidepressant SSRIs tend to work well with these people. Add SAMe at 400 mg a day – watch for depression or anxiety.

12. <u>Overmethylator</u> (Low Histamine Level) – SAMe makes people suicidal – DO NOT GIVE/TAKE to ANYONE who is an overmethylator! You should give/take folate or folinic acid instead. Plus SSRI's are bad for these people. (AND ALSO, SSRIs ARE NOT FOR KIDS WITH ASD). If you are depressed use a TCA (tri-cyclic anti-depressant) such as low dose amitryptiline at night (25 mg).

13. Add folinic acid – start low (220 mcg? Cut the folinic acid tablet in fourths) and go very slow. Take no more than 2 per day but work your way higher if need be or helps.

14. Try Vitamin C. One a day is sufficient (unless your SpectraCell™ Micronutrient Panel shows you need more).

15. Add niacin at 25 mg a day in multiple doses for nausea or anxiety. Again start with one and maybe if needed add another. Use your SpectraCell™ Micronutrient panel as a guide. You can go as high as 6 per day.

16. Start with a natural whole food multivitamin at one per day (one capsule or tablet or packet, if chosen correctly, is the easiest and most natural way to get a TINY AMOUNT OF NATURAL FOLATE IN).

17. Add fish oil – no matter what the front of the bottle says, your goal is to get 2500 mg/day of EPA and DHA – start with one per day (with meals) and after a few weeks go to twice a day (to prevent clotting and strokes and other thrombotic events).

18. Add probiotics -- 2 in the morning or two at night – take with food.

19. If you have any clotting risk (check with your doctor) add nattokinase (2,000 Fu), to reduce clotting risk naturally.

20. After 1-2 weeks, if no nausea, add or start on Folinic Acid 500 mcg (try half of one per day).

21. After two weeks with no problems (nausea, aches, pains, etc.) add your chosen "methylation support" capsule as a I outlined at one per day. Take first thing in the morning.

22. NOTE: Homozygous A1298C patients will not get the same really great results from the "methylation support" capsule. Though they do benefit from taking them.

23. After one week increase the "methylation support" capsule to two per day.

24. After another week and no problems (i.e. flu-like symptoms), go to three per day (2 in AM and 1 at lunch).

25. Nauseated or feel funky? Add NIACIN at 25 mg a dose (watch for flushing – just a weird side effect). Take up to 6 per day (they're safe but you just may flush which can be misery).

26. Is your Whole Blood Histamine level **high**? You are an **"undermethylator"**. Start with methionine 200 or 250 mg capsules first. If two each day are well tolerated then change to SAMe (and avoid extra methylfolate or especially folic acid!).

27. Is your Whole Blood Histamine level **low**? You are an **"overmethylator"**. Then add B12 500 mcg slowly climbing to 1-3 per day – but do it SLOWLY.

28. After a few weeks and feeling the benefits (you will) please take an extra "methylation support" capsule at noon before lunch or with lunch (so now you're on 4/day).

29. After a few more weeks try 5 "methylation support" capsules per day (3 in AM and 2 at lunch). If nausea or flu-like problems back it back down to three or four per day.

30. Keep going up on the "methylation support" capsule until you hit 8. That will be your dose. Forever.

31. WARNING! If you ever miss or stop taking your "methylation support" capsule you will probably feel pretty horrible pretty quickly (a day or two into it?). If you don't believe, try it and see for your self. You crash back to how you used to feel pretty fast. It is not good. DO NOT STOP YOUR "methylation support" capsule.

32. Add other vitamins as needed according to the SpectraCell® Results.

33. Add 5-HTP at night but just a tiny dose (50 mg). Helps with sleep and anxiety. Might only work temporarily. To learn more and to get another perspective – none of this is easy.)

34. For joint inflammation or arthritis pain use Thorne Research Meriva-SR™ 1-2 per day (hat tip to Dr. Victoria Sucher for this great pointer).

35. For ICS pain/inflammation try Thorne Research AR Encaps™[81] 2 per day (but start on 1 as a test).

36. Add SAMe at 400 mg a day – watch for depression or anxiety. One per day is usually sufficient (but like I have advised try methionine 500 mg capsules first).

37. CoQ10 could also be helpful – especially if your Spectracell™ Micronutrient Panel suggests it. My preferred Coq10 is ubiquinol 200 mg a day.

38. TMG is another option.

39. Add BH4 to your diet if you think you need (see Genova™ testing above) or cannot bring it up natural. Keep in mind it's expensive and hard to get. Get Pteridin-4 at $79.50 for 60 capsules of 2.5mg BH4 – so a month's worth (4/day) would be two bottles or 120 capsules. (It may not be available.) *http://www.spectrum-*

supplements.com/tetrahydrobiopterin-60-capsules.html

40. Repeat your lab testing on a regular basis – especially the SpectraCell™ Comprehensive Panel and Whole Blood Histamine levels.

41. HOMOZYGOUS A1298C patients are my most difficult to treat. They really suffer. Most of their issues are just abject depression. Can be a lot of mental stuff.

42. If you're in the 50% who do not feel better be patient. Look to see if you're an under or over-methylator. See if you need methionine first then try SAMe. Also, if you're anxious try GABA (500-600 mg at night) or 5-HTP to help you sleep. Or try TMG too. See if that helps. You have many options. DO NOT GIVE UP!

RESOURCES

HEARTFIXER: A GREAT WEBSITE on METHYL CYCLE NUTRIGENOMICS

(Search NUTRAHACKER on his page and upload your 23andme DNA® data to that website then get your evaluation report from HEARTFIXER.)

http://www.heartfixer.com/AMRI-Nutrigenomics.htm

Another site is Stanford's Interpretome®:

http://interpretome.com/

The best possibly for 23andme DNA results interpretations might be:

http://www.23andyou.com/3rdparty

21

DIAGNOSIS PROTOCOL SUMMARIZED

HERE ARE THE steps I'd take you through if you came to my office:

1.) If you suspect that you might have MTHFR, start with basic labs and hormone panels – you can go to my website to download the panels I suggest (and order them yourself if your doctor won't help) – *danpursermd.com* you'd have to pay for these labs yourself as it's a self-order lab site, but at least you don't have to beg some doctor to order them for you (this lab has 1,300 draw sites nationwide and is really inexpensive). I want to see what's being affected. Make sure you add a HOMOCYSTEINE level.

2.)   I'd also suggest a SpectraCell™ Comprehensive Micronutrient Panel to determine which vitamins are deficient – this can give you or your physician HUGE direction as to what's going on.

3.)   If you strongly suspect that MTHFR is the correct root cause diagnosis and while your doctor has a needle in your arm for the labs and SpectraCell™ MicroNutrient panel, ask him to get a SpectraCell™ MTHFR lab. Easy.

4.)   Three to four weeks later (it takes that long to get results) you and your physician need to go through these labs and see where the problems lie.

Go by the vitamin deficiencies and "borderline" deficiencies on your SpectraCell™ Micronutrient panel first. You have to deal with those deficiencies, but they will guide you too.

If you have a bunch of B vitamin deficiencies then MTHFR becomes a big (ger) possibility.

5.)   Look at your hormones – if they're oddly low this could be a reflection of either the vitamin deficiencies or the MTHFR mutations you might have.

6.)   Get on the right diet and get the book – either GAPS™ or Spectrum™ (by Ornish) or a "low methionine" vegetarian diet.

7.)   Next look at the MTHFR testing – do you have any defects? If you have a MTHFR mutation but are heterozygous (just one SNP which stands for Single Nucleotide Polymorphism) and have any deficiencies, deal with it accordingly – HOMOCYSTEINE SUPREME® may work fine for you. Press your dose up to 2 in the morning and one at noon – hold there – if there is any nausea, back it up.

8.)   You can add SAM-E (rarely) or NIACIN CRT™ (again just for any nausea or niacin deficiency noted on the Micronutrient panel) just take them in small amounts or moderation.

9.)   After 90 days it's time to repeat everything. Yep, you get to give another blood donation (that YOU pay for!), to see what improvement you've had, but hopefully by 90 days you're feeling better and better. I've seen patients be shocked at how good they get. So hope and pray for that level of improvement.

10.)   Keep up the good work. Get the Micronutrient panel at least annually for the rest of your life. Also repeat your histamine, homocysteine, and urinary pyrrole levels – they should all be normal. Energy levels should be "normal" at this time (which the patient/you should love). Any non-recovery needs to be drilled deeper.

11.)   Have a great life! Read on for freebies and downloads I offer my readers.

THE "UNDERMETHYLATOR" MTHFR WOMAN GETS HAPPY

She was smiling. Her hair was fixed. She had brighter color on.

I sat down across from her. "How are you doing?"

"Great! I feel amazing!"

"What are you taking? Is it legal?"

She laughed – a new sound from her. "Hope so. It's that SAMe you gave me – it's amazing. Taking 3 a day. And the OptiZinc™ - taking 5 a day. Best I've ever felt. I never imagined…"

I smiled. "You can try some more SAMe. It all just gets better from here."

She laughed. "I can't imagine."

ONE FINAL NOTE

Wow, you're done. But hopefully we're not done. This book will be ever evolving just as the field of epigenetics is evolving – Dr's Ben Lynch, Jill Carnahan and other forerunners will keep coming up with new info and so will I. This field is soooo new we have to evolve or die.

Thanks for taking the time to read this book. I hope it helped.

If you enjoyed the read – if it's helped your life in some small way then would you please leave me a review on this book wherever you bought it? Just consider it part of paying it forward so the next reader might be encouraged to take a moment to improve their knowledge, their existence, and their life.

Go here to find this book:

http://www/greatmedebooks.com

And again, thanks so much for taking the time to learn this material and to spend it with me.

ADDENDUM A

A METHYLATIONS PATHWAY MAP[82]

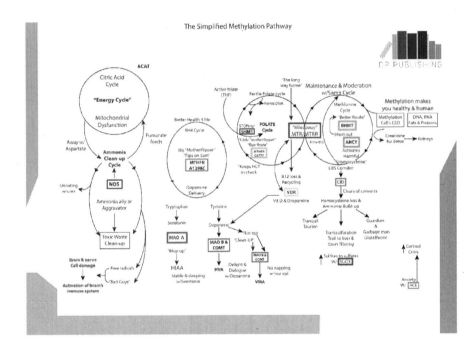

The Simplified Methylation Pathway

ADDENDUM B

WEBSITES AND OTHER RESOURCES

http://mthfrliving.com/

https://www.23andme.com/

http://23andyou/3rdparty/

http://www.stopthethyroidmadness.com/mthfr/

http://mthfr.net/ - probably one of THE best resources on MTHFR

Walsh Research Institute's YouTube Channel – full of incredible information on the MTHFR enzyme issues – Dr. William Walsh is a master of epigenetics and biochemistry research behind most of these enzyme deficiencies - *https://www.youtube.com/channel/UC6tEkmE3CoHnCbfgWP EpPcA*

Also *http://walshinstitute.org*

GREAT website with outreach clinics listed – Dr. Mensah is another medical genius with MTHFR issues and treatment and has clinics in Illinois and around the country. *http://www.mensahmedical.com/resourcecenter.html*

http://ghr.nlm.nih.gov/gene/MTHFR - *National Library of Medicine*

http://catalog.designsforhealth.com/SAMe

http://catalog.designsforhealth.com/Homocysteine-Supreme

http://catalog.designsforhealth.com/Niacin-CRT-60

http://www.realgsh.com

http://gapsdiet.com

http://dramyneuzil.com/tag/mthfr/

http://www.integratedhealthblog.com

⸮

APPENDIX C

PROTOCOL FOR HETEROZYGOUS MTHFR

1. Begin by seeing your doctor – make sure he understands biochemistry regarding MTHFR. Lay out your symptoms and what you think.

2. Then start with a 1) SpectraCell™ Comprehensive Micronutrient Panel, 2) Homocysteine Level, 3) Histamine Level.

3. Try Homocysteine Supreme™ if your Spectracell Metabolic panel suggests you need it. Also cover any other vitamins.

4. If suggestive on the Metabolic Panel (when it returns) then get the Spectracell™ MTHFR testing done and 23andme™ done too.

5. Look at your WHOLE BLOOD HISTAMINE LEVEL – you need to know your status – remember to have it drawn when they first check your Homocysteine level.

6. (REMEMBER - if Whole Blood Histamine is LOW, the individual will be overmethylated. And if it is HIGH, they will be undermethylated.)

7. Undermethylator (High Histamine Level) – Try a trial of methionine 500 mg capsules first (up to two day) then if there are no problems, change to SAMe -- which really works for these! It makes most people happy! But don't give any folate/folic acid! Also, antidepressant SSRIs tend to work well with these people.

8. Overmethylator (Low Histamine Level <40 ng/ml) – SAMe makes most patients suicidal – DO NOT GIVE/TAKE this if you are a overmethylator! Give/take folate instead. Plus, SSRI's are bad for these people.

9. Add MethylFolate (L-5-MTHF) or add SAMe according to your histamine status.

10. Repeat all three tests above on a regular basis.

APPENDIX D

PROTOCOL FOR HOMOZYGOUS C677T

(This is just a path – it may have to be set aside – do not go down it blindly – be careful and be correctable.)

HOMOZYGOUS C677T PROTOCOL© BY DAN PURSER M.D.

1.   Get SpectraCell© Comprehensive Micronutrient Panel - critical, and saves a ton of money on enzyme testing.

2.   Get Whole Blood Histamine Level – helps determine methylation status.

3.   Get your Homocysteine Level – determines inflammation status and treatment value.

4.   Start with a natural whole food multivitamin at one per day (one capsule or tablet or packet, if chosen correctly, is the easiest and most natural way to get a TINY AMOUNT OF NATURAL FOLATE IN).

5.   Add fish oil – no matter what the front of the bottle says, your goal is to get 2500 mg/day of EPA and DHA – start with one per day (with meals) and after a few weeks go to twice a day (to prevent clotting and strokes and other thrombotic events)

6.   Add probiotics -- 2 in the morning or two at night – take with food.

7.   If you have any clotting risk (check with your doctor) add nattokinase (2,000 Fu), to reduce clotting risk naturally.

8.   After 1-2 weeks, if no nausea, add or start on Folinic Acid 500 mcg (try half of one per day)

9.   After two weeks with no problems (nausea, aches, pains, etc.) add your chosen "methylation support" capsule as a I outlined at one per day. Take first thing in the morning.

10. On the third week increase the "methylation support" capsule to two per day.

11. After another week and no problems (i.e. flu-like symptoms), go to three per day (2 in AM and 1 at lunch).

12. Nauseated or feel funky? Add NIACIN at 25 mg a dose (watch for flushing – just a weird side effect). Take up to 6 per day (they're safe but you just may flush which can be misery).

13. Is your Whole Blood Histamine level **high**? You are an "**undermethylator**". Start with methionine 200 or 250 mg capsules first. If two each day are well tolerated then change to SAMe (and avoid extra methylfolate or especially folic acid!).

14. Is your Whole Blood Histamine level **low**? You are an "**overmethylator**". Then add B12 500 mcg slowly climbing to 1-3 per day – but do it SLOWLY.

15. After a few weeks of feeling the benefits (you will), take an extra "methylation support" capsule at noon before lunch or with lunch (so now you're on 4/day).

16. After a few more weeks try 5 "methylation support" capsules per day (3 in AM and 2 at lunch). If nausea or flu-like problems back it back down to three or four per day.

17. Keep going up on the "methylation support" capsule until you hit 8. That will be your dose. Forever.

18. WARNING! If you ever miss or stop taking your "methylation support" capsule you will probably feel pretty horrible pretty quickly (a day or two into it?). If you don't believe try it and see for your self. You crash back to how you used to feel pretty fast. It is not good. DO NOT STOP YOUR "methylation support" capsule.

19. Add other vitamins as needed according to the SpectraCell® Results.

20. Don't forget to add Niacin (25 mg) or B6 (25 mg -- in the form of hydroxycobalamin) if nausea occurs.

21. What should you feel now? Welcome to normalcy. You should feel TONS of ENERGY. Your testosterone or other hormones (unless you're in menopause) should be slowly rising after 3-4 months – eventually to a much more normal level. It becomes very obvious if we dialed it all in correctly. This approach should work for about 90% of C677T people but for some it will not – so see your doctor or naturopath if it does not.

22. If you're in the 10% who do not feel better be patient. Look to see if you're an under or over-methylator. See if you need methionine first then try SAMe. Also, if you're anxious try GABA (500-600 mg at night) or 5-HTP to help you sleep. Or try TMG too. See if that helps. You have many options. DO NOT GIVE UP!

APPENDIX E

PROTOCOL FOR HOMOZYGOUS A1298C

(This is just a path – it may have to be set aside – do not go down it blindly – be careful and ne correctable.)

Hard to make a stepwise approach to this so please understand this is just a rough attempt at this that I hope some of you will find helpful. I also cannot factor in everyone's finances so I'm assuming everyone has the money to do all of this – I am sorry if you don't - truly.

Signs? Symptoms? Conditions? Do these all match MTHFR especially the Homozygous A1298C variant?

1. Get a Spectracell™ Comprehensive Micronutrient Panel – this is INTRACELLULAR so incredibly accurate - get this from a doctor who is signed up as a Spectracell™ provider. Carefully treat the deficiencies (see examples in this chapter) with the proper vitamins and supplements for your condition.

2. Also add a Homocysteine Level, and Whole Blood Histamine Level (to determine methylation capabilities).

3. Get a Metametrix™ or Genova™ Biopterin/Neopterin Urine panel – very helpful to se where you're at in spectrum.

4. Get a Genova™ ION™ Profile with 40 Amino Acids – helps to detail what else might be going on. This could come in very handy later.

5. Obtain and perform a salivary http://23andme.com genetic profile on yourself so you know what other mutations and enzymes you just might have. If this is the case, please go to the great website http://www.23andyou.com/3rdparty or use *Genetic Genie* which is free (leave a donation to their Paypal™ account please so they keep offering their valuable compilation service)to get an interpretation site you like. Or see RESOURCE in this chapter.

6. Assuming your Homozygous for A1298C, tighten your diet with the amount of protein you ingest (see this calculator website to determine your allowable RDA for protein).

7. Add Moderately High Purine foods to your diet too (see list) such as Asparagus, Bacon, Beef, Cauliflower, Chicken, Chicken soup, Crab, Ham, Kidney beans, Lamb, Lentils, Lima beans, Lobster, Mushrooms, Mutton, Navy beans, Oatmeal, Peas, Pork, Salmon, Sheep, Spinach, Trout, Tuna, Turkey, etc.

8. Add broad spectrum light therapy daily for 15-20 minutes – start low and build-up slowly. In the depths of winter go longer if need be. I and my patients like this light the best off Amazon™ - Lightphoria™ 10,000LUX Energy Light Lamp from Sphere Gadget Technologie.

9. (REMEMBER - if Whole Blood Histamine is LOW, the individual will be overmethylated. And if it is HIGH, they will be undermethylated.)

10. ★(FOR KIDS WITH ASD) Undermethylator (High Whole Blood Histamine Level >70 ng/ml) – SAMe works for these! Makes them happy (but start on methionine trial first 200-500 mg). DO NOT give folate/folic acid! Also antidepressant SSRIs tend to work well with these people. Add SAMe at 400 mg a day – watch for depression or anxiety.

11. Overmethylator (Low Histamine Level) – SAMe makes suicidal – DO NOT GIVE/TAKE! Give/take folate or folinic acid instead. Plus SSRI's are bad for these people. (AND ALSO, SSRIs NOT FOR KIDS WITH ASD). If depressed use a TCA (tri-cyclic anti-depressant) such as low dose amitryptiline at night (25 mg).

12. Add folinic acid – start low (220 mcg? Cut the folinic acid tablet in fourths) and go very slow. Take no more than 2 per day but work your way higher if need be or helps.

13. Try Vitamin C. One a day is sufficient (unless your SpectraCell™ Micronutrient Panel shows you need more).

14. Add niacin at 25 mg a day in multiple doses for nausea or anxiety. Again start with one and maybe if needed add another. Use your SpectraCell™ Micronutrient panel as a guide. Can go as high as 6 per day.

15. Start with a natural whole food multivitamin at one per day (one capsule or tablet or packet, if chosen correctly, is the easiest and most natural way to get a TINY AMOUNT OF NATURAL FOLATE IN).

16. Add fish oil – no matter what the front of the bottle says, your goal is to get 2500 mg/day of EPA and DHA – start with one per day (with meals) and after a few weeks go to twice a day (to prevent clotting and strokes and other thrombotic events).

17. Add probiotics -- 2 in the morning or two at night – take with food.

18. If you have any clotting risk (check with your doctor) add nattokinase (2,000 Fu), to reduce clotting risk naturally.

19. After 1-2 weeks, if no nausea, add or start on Folinic Acid 500 mcg (try half of one per day).

20. After two weeks with no problems (nausea, aches, pains, etc.) add your chosen "methylation support" capsule as a I outlined at one per day. Take first thing in the morning.

21. NOTE: Homozygous A1298C patients will not get the same really great results from the "methylation support" capsule. Though they do benefit from taking them.

22. After one week increase the "methylation support" capsule to two per day.

23. After another week and no problems (i.e. flu-like symptoms), go to three per day (2 in AM and 1 at lunch).

24. Nauseated or feel funky? Add NIACIN at 25 mg a dose (watch for flushing – just a weird side effect). Take up to 6 per day (they're safe but you just may flush which can be misery).

25. Is your Whole Blood Histamine level **high**? You are an **"undermethylator"**. Start with methionine 200 or 250 mg capsules first. If two each day are well tolerated then change to SAMe (and avoid extra methylfolate or especially folic acid!).

26. Is your Whole Blood Histamine level **low**? You are an **"overmethylator"**. Then add B12 500 mcg slowly climbing to 1-3 per day – but do it SLOWLY.

27. After a few weeks and feeling the benefits (you will) please take an extra "methylation support" capsule at noon before lunch or with lunch (so now you're on 4/day).

28. After a few more weeks try 5 "methylation support" capsules per day (3 in AM and 2 at lunch). If nausea or flu-like problems back it back down to three or four per day.

29. Keep going up on the "methylation support" capsule until you hit 8. That will be your dose. Forever.

30. WARNING! If you ever miss or stop taking your "methylation support" capsule you will probably feel pretty horrible pretty quickly (a day or two into it?). If you don't believe try it and see for your self. You crash back to how you used to feel pretty fast. It is not good. DO NOT STOP YOUR "methylation support" capsule.

31. Add other vitamins as needed according to the SpectraCell® Results.

32. Add 5-HTP at night but just a tiny dose (50 mg). Helps with sleep and anxiety. Might only work temporarily. To learn more and to get another perspective – none of this is easy.)

33. For joint inflammation or arthritis pain use Thorne Research Meriva-SR™ 1-2 per day (hat tip to Dr. Victoria Sucher for this great pointer).

34. For ICS pain/inflammation try Thorne Research AR Encaps™[83] 2 per day (but start on 1 as a test).

35. Add SAMe at 400 mg a day – watch for depression or anxiety. One per day is usually sufficient (but like I have advised try methionine 500 mg capsules first).

36. CoQ10 could also be helpful – especially if your Spectracell™ Micronutrient Panel suggests it. My preferred Coq10 is ubiquinol 200 mg a day.

37. TMG is another option.

38. Add BH4 to your diet if you think you need (see Genova™ testing above) or cannot bring it up natural. Keep in mind it's expensive and hard to get. Get Pteridin-4 at $79.50 for 60 capsules of 2.5mg BH4 – so a month's worth (4/day) would be two bottles or 120 capsules. (It may not be available.) ***http://www.spectrum-supplements.com/tetrahydrobiopterin-60-capsules.html***

39. Repeat your lab testing on a regular basis – especially the SpectraCell™ Comprehensive Panel and Whole Blood Histamine levels.

40. HOMOZYGOUS A1298C patients are my most difficult to treat. They really suffer. Most of their issues are just abject depression. Can be a lot of mental stuff.

41. If you're in the 50% who do not feel better be patient. Look to see if you're an under or over-methylator. See if you need methionine first then try SAMe. Also, if you're anxious try GABA (500-600 mg at night) or 5-HTP to help you sleep. Or try TMG too. See if that helps. You have many options. DO NOT GIVE UP!

Why Did I Call This Book The 85% Solution?

I've been asked a number of times why I named this book the way I did.

Studies have shown that among fair-haired blue eyed populations (i.e. of northern European descent) that MTHFR prevalence could be as high as 85%. And in Utah where I live this is the predominant population – northern European. Also fair haired (Castillian) Spaniards have a high incidence also (almost 85%).

There are also a great deal of Scottish, Irish and British subjects descended from Vikings (Danish and Norwegian) and so they also have a very high incidence – and great number of their offspring live in Utah due to proselytizing by the LDS Church in England, the British Isles in the 19th century.

I also always write my books first as patient handouts and educational pieces (and still use them that way even after printing) thus the writing and birth of this book. Thanks for the interest and to all of you who've read this – I hoped it's helped in some small way.

--Dan Purser MD

Supplement Recommendations

NUTRAscriptives®

They have a fairly comprehensive line of products to treat MTHFR. They are my preferred provider in terms of both quality and variety as they are one of the few that carry most everything you will need.

Their products include:

MTHFR Main Support

Copper Support

B12/Folate

GABA

Methyl Folate

SAM-e

Zinc Picolinate

Calcium Folinate

www.nutrascriptives.com

Attribution:

I want to thank Kerri Daly for all of her hard work and knowledge in this area -- many ideas in this book would have not been possible without her suggestions and intelligence. Thank you Kerri!

danpursermd.com

BIG REMINDER:

Please leave a short review if you enjoyed this book. Thanks!

WANT TO CONNECT WITH DR. PURSER?

MEN:

> To download THREE FREE REPORTS full of helpful MEN's information on testosterone issues and other medical problems and as a BONUS my DR PURSER LAB SOLUTIONS REPORT just clink on the link here:

http://www.drpursergift.com

> For Dr. Purser's Amazon Author Page linking to all of his books (including his five #1 books):

http://www.greatmedebooks.com

> To get to know Dr. Purser better and to get his email newsletter (full of discounts and coupons and freebies):

danpursermd.com

WOMEN:

> For WOMEN's information on their health issues (PMS, migraines, endometriosis, menopause, thyroid, and osteoporosis) and a more thoughtful approach to those problems:

danpursermd.com

> To download THREE FREE REPORTS full of helpful WOMEN's information on testosterone issues and other medical problems and as a BONUS my DR PURSER LAB SOLUTIONS REPORT just clink on the link here:

Facebook: Dan Purser M.D.

Twitter: @danpursermd

Pinterest: Dan Purser MD

Endnotes

1   No author listed. Accessed 13 May 2015 online at
    http://www.gbhealthwatch.com/GND-Cardiovascular-Diseases-MTHFR.php

2   Osian G, Procopciuc L, et al. C677T and A1298C mutations in the MTHFR gene
    and survival in colorectal cancer. J Gastrointestin Liver Dis. 2009
    Dec;18(4):455-60

3   No   author   listed.   Accessed   9   September   2015   at
    http://report.nih.gov/NIHfactsheets/ViewFactSheet.aspx?csid=45&key=H#H
4 No author listed. Accessed 13 May 2015 online at
    http://ghr.nlm.nih.gov/gene/MTHFR

5   Bowthorpe,   J.   Accessed   10   June   2015   online   at
    http://www.stopthethyroidmadness.com/mthfr/
6 No author listed. Accessed 12 May 2015 online at http://MTHFR.net

7   Carnahan,   J.   Accessed   12   May   2015   online   at
    http://www.jillcarnahan.com/2014/02/23/health-tips-for-anyone-with-a-
    mthfr-gene-mutation/
8   Carnahan,   J.   Accessed   12   May   2015   online   at
    http://www.jillcarnahan.com/2014/02/23/health-tips-for-anyone-with-a-
    mthfr-gene-mutation/
9 No author listed. Accessed 12 May 2015 online at
    http://www.stopthethyroidmadness.com/mthfr/

10 Slooter AJ, Rosendaal FR, et al. Prothrombotic conditions, oral contraceptives,
    and the risk of ischemic stroke. J Thromb Haemost. 2005 Jun;3(6):1213-7

11 No author listed. Accessed 13 May 2015 online at

http://www.gbhealthwatch.com/GND-Cardiovascular-Diseases-MTHFR.php

[12] No author listed. Accessed 13 May 2015 online at
http://www.rockwellnutrition.com/p-homocysteine-supreme-60-caps-by-designs-for-health#.VVNsAtNVhHw

[13] Eleftheriadou I, Grigoropoulou P, et al. The effect of hyperhomocysteinemia on aortic distensibility in healthy individuals. Nutrition. 2013 Jun;29(6):876-80. doi: 10.1016/j.nut.2012.12.026.

[14] Tuncer SK, Kaldirim U, et al. Neopterin, homocysteine, and ADMA levels during and after urticaria attack. Turk J Med Sci. 2015;45(6):1251-5.

[15] No author listed. Accessed 12 May 2015 online at
http://www.rockwellnutrition.com/designs-for-health-supplements-homocysteine-supreme-120-caps.html#.VVLBvtNVhHw

[16] Laboratory Evaluations in Molecular Medicine. Alexander Brally, PhD, CCN and Richard Lord, PhD (Metametrix Biochemistry Textbook)

[17] Catargi B, Parrot-Roulaud F, Cochet C, Ducassou D, Roger P, Tabarin A. Homocysteine, hypothyroidism, and effect of thyroid hormone replacement. Thyroid. 1999 Dec;9(12):1163-6

[18] Homocysteine Lowering Trialists' Collaboration. Dose-dependent effects of folic acid on blood concentrations of homocysteine: a meta-analysis of the randomized trials. Am J Clin Nutr. 2005 Oct;82(4):806-12

[19] Evers S et al. Features, symptoms and neurophysiological findings in stroke associated with hyperhomocysteinemia. Arch Neurol 1997;54:1276-82

[20] Berlin H BR, and Brante G. Oral treatment of pernicious anemia with high doses of vitamin B12 without intrinisic factor. Acta Med Scand. 1968; 184:247-248

[21] Stern LL, Bagley PJ, Rosenberg IH, Selhub J. Conversion of 5-formyltetrahydrofolic acid to 5-methyltetrahydrofolic acid is unimpaired in folate-adequate persons homozygous for the C677T mutation in the methylenetetrahydrofolate reductase gene. J Nutr. 2000 Sep;130(9):2238-42

[22] Kelly GS. Folates: supplemental forms and therapeutic applications. Altern Med Rev. 1998 Jun;3(3):208-20

[23] Bayes B, Pastor MC, Bonal J, Junca J, Romero R. Homocysteine and lipid

peroxidation in haemodialysis: role of folinic acid and vitamin E. Nephrol Dial Transplant. 2001 Nov;16(11):2172-5

[24] Laboratory Evaluations in Molecular Medicine J. Alexander Brally, PhD, CCN and Richard Lord, PhD (Metametrix Biochemistry Textbook)

[25] Laboratory Evaluations in Molecular Medicine J. Alexander Brally, PhD, CCN and Richard Lord, PhD (Metametrix Biochemistry Textbook)

[26] Wilson, L. Trimethylglycine or TMG. Accessed 05 Aug 2015 at http://www.drlwilson.com/ARTICLES/TRIMTHYLGLYCINE.htm © August 2014, The Center For Development

[27] Wilson, L. Trimethylglycine or TMG. Accessed 05 Aug 2015 at http://www.drlwilson.com/ARTICLES/TRIMTHYLGLYCINE.htm © August 2014, The Center For Development

[28] No author listed. Accessed 13 May 2015 online at http://www.rockwellnutrition.com/L-5-MTHF-Capsules-by-Designs-For-Health.html#.VVLEW9NVhHw

[29] Neuzil, A. Accessed 14 May 2015 online at http://dramyneuzil.com/tag/mthfr/

[30] Myers, A. Accessed online 17 June 2015 at http://www.mindbodygreen.com/0-11175/everything-you-need-to-know-about-histamine-intolerance.html

[31] Myers, A. Accessed online 17 June 2015 at http://www.mindbodygreen.com/0-11175/everything-you-need-to-know-about-histamine-intolerance.html

[32] Myers, A. Accessed online 17 June 2015 at http://www.mindbodygreen.com/0-11175/everything-you-need-to-know-about-histamine-intolerance.html

[33] Tsafrir, J. Accessed online 17 June 2015 at http://primaldocs.com/members-blog/histamine-methylation-and-mthfr/

[34] Tsafrir, J. Accessed online 17 June 2015 at http://primaldocs.com/members-blog/histamine-methylation-and-mthfr/

35 Walsh, WJ. Accessed online 17 June 2015 at
http://www.mensahmedical.com/images/Depression_PP_2.pdf

36 Walsh, WJ. Accessed online 17 June 2015 at
http://www.mensahmedical.com/images/Depression_PP_2.pdf

37 Walsh, WJ. Accessed online 17 June 2015 at
http://www.mensahmedical.com/images/Depression_PP_2.pdf
38 Walsh, WJ. Accessed online 17 June 2015 at
http://www.mensahmedical.com/images/Depression_PP_2.pdf

39 Walsh, WJ. Accessed online 17 June 2015 at
http://www.mensahmedical.com/images/Depression_PP_2.pdf

40 Walsh, WJ. Accessed online 17 June 2015 at
http://www.mensahmedical.com/images/Depression_PP_2.pdf

41 Carnahan, J. Accessed online 17 June 2015 at
http://doccarnahan.blogspot.com/2013/11/histamine-intolerance-could-this-be.html

42 Tsafrir, J. Accessed online 17 June 2015 at http://primaldocs.com/members-blog/histamine-methylation-and-mthfr/

43 Tsafrir, J. Accessed online 17 June 2015 at http://primaldocs.com/members-blog/histamine-methylation-and-mthfr/

44 No author listed. Accessed 12 May 2015 online at
https://pgenpt.wordpress.com/2014/06/23/trying-out-sam-e-smart-people-can-do-dumb-things/

45 SHOMON, M. Accessed 12 May 2015 online at
http://thyroid.about.com/od/MTHFR-Gene-Mutations-and-Polymorphisms/fl/The-Link-Between-MTHFR-Gene-Mutations-and-Disease-Including-Thyroid-Health.htm

46 No author listed. Accessed 13 May 2015 online at
http://catalog.designsforhealth.com/SAMe

47 Neuzil, A. Accessed 14 May 2015 online at
http://dramyneuzil.com/tag/mthfr.

48 Neuzil, A. Accessed 14 May 2015 online at
http://dramyneuzil.com/tag/mthfr.

[49] Aw TY, Wierzbicka G, Jones DP. "Oral glutathione increases tissue glutathione in vivo", Chemico-Biological Interactions, 1991;80(1):89-97.

[50] Hagen TM, Wierzbicka GT et al. "Bioavailability of dietary glutathione: effect on plasma concentration", The American Journal of Physiology, 1990 Oct; 259(4 Pt 1):G524-9.

[51] No author listed. Accessed April 1, 2016 at https://www.novapublishers.com/catalog/product_info.php?products_id=42434.

[52] No author listed. Accessed April 1, 2016 at http://www.essentialgsh.com/glutathione.html.

[53] No author listed. Accessed 13 May 2015 online at http://www.gbhealthwatch.com/GND-Cardiovascular-Diseases-MTHFR.php

[54] No author listed. Accessed 13 May 2015 online at http://www.stopthethyroidmadness.com/mthfr/

[55] No author listed. Accessed 1 August 2015 at http://www.whfoods.com/genpage.php?tname=george&dbid=51

[56] No author listed. Accessed 1 August 2015 at http://www.whfoods.com/genpage.php?tname=george&dbid=51

[57] Hotamisligil GS, Breakefield XO (Aug 1991). "Human monoamine oxidase A gene determines levels of enzyme activity". American Journal of Human Genetics 49 (2): 383–92. PMC 1683299. PMID 1678250.

[58] Grimsby J, Chen K, Wang LJ, Lan NC, Shih JC (May 1991). "Human monoamine oxidase A and B genes exhibit identical exon-intron organization". Proceedings of the National Academy of Sciences of the United States of America 88 (9): 3637–41. doi:10.1073/pnas.88.9.3637. PMC 51507. PMID 2023912.

[59] Rosenberg S, Templeton AR, et al. The association of DNA sequence variation at the MAOA genetic locus with quantitative behavioural traits in normal males. Hum Genet. 2006 Nov;120(4):447-59.

[60] http://redmountainclinic.com/

[61] Rostenberg. A Genetic Cause of Pain and Anxiety – COMT, MAO and MTHFR. Accessed 09 August 2015 online at http://beyondmthfr.com/2014/11/04/a-genetic-cause-of-pain-and-anxiety-comt-mao-and-mthfr/

[62] Rostenberg. A Genetic Cause of Pain and Anxiety – COMT, MAO and MTHFR. Accessed 09 August 2015 online at http://beyondmthfr.com/2014/11/04/a-genetic-cause-of-pain-and-anxiety-comt-mao-and-mthfr/

[63] Gondawandaland. Accessed 09 August 2015 online at http://forums.phoenixrising.me/index.php?threads/comt-methylfolate-or-folic-acid.37477/

[64] Luine VN, Rhodes JC. Gonadal hormone regulation of MAO and other enzymes in hypothalamic areas. Neuroendocrinology. 1983;36(3):235-41.

[65] Cowan LD, Gordis L, et al. Breast cancer incidence in women with a history of progesterone deficiency. Am J Epidemiol. 1981 Aug;114(2):209-17.

[66] Johnson, D. Accessed 09 August 2015 online at http://mthfralliance.com/2014/02/03/why-b6-is-the-queen-b/

[67] No author listed. Accessed 09 August 2015 online at http://mthfrliving.com/health-tips/supplementing-for-mthfr-b12/

[68] No author listed. "MedLine Plus: Pernicious Anemia" Accessed 09 August 2015 online at http://www.nlm.nih.gov/medlineplus/ency/article/000569.htm

[69] Scott JM, Weir DG. The methyl folate trap. A physiological response in man to prevent methyl group deficiency in kwashiorkor (methionine deficiency) and an explanation for folic-acid induced exacerbation of subacute combined degeneration in pernicious anaemia. Lancet. 1981 Aug 15;2(8242):337-40

[70] Lynch, B Accessed 09 August 2015 online at http://mthfr.net/methylfolate-taking-too-much-a-problem/2012/01/08/

[71] No author listed. Accessed 1 August 2015 at http://www.detoxpuzzle.com/bh4.php

[72] Diagnosis, treatment and follow-up of patients with tetrahydrobiopterin deficiency in Shandong province, China. Brain Dev. 2015 Jun;37(6):592-8. doi: 10.1016/j.braindev.2014.09.008

[73] Hoekstra R, Fekkes D, et al. Effect of light therapy on biopterin, neopterin and

tryptophan in patients with seasonal affective disorder. Psychiatry Res. 2003 Aug 30;120(1):37-42

[74] No author listed. Accessed 1 August 2015 at https://en.wikipedia.org/wiki/Guanosine_triphosphate

[75] No author listed. Accessed 31 July 2015 online at http://forums.phoenixrising.me/index.php?threads/x-men-mutant-protocols-a1298c-homozygous.22067/

[76] Carnahan, J. Accessed 1 August 2015 at http://www.integratedhealthblog.com/supplementing-with-folate-coenzymes-5-mthf-and-folinic-acid/

[77] Carnahan, J. Accessed 1 August 2015 at http://www.integratedhealthblog.com/supplementing-with-folate-coenzymes-5-mthf-and-folinic-acid/

[78] Carnahan, J. Accessed 18 June 2015 online at http://www.jillcarnahan.com/2014/02/23/health-tips-for-anyone-with-a-mthfr-gene-mutation

[79] I. Smith, K. Hyland, et al. Clinical Role of Pteridine Therapy in Tetrahydrobiopterin Deficiency. Inherited Disorders of Vitamins and Cofactors 1985, pp 39-45

[80] Purchase at http://www.spectrum-supplements.com/tetrahydrobiopterin-60-capsules.html

[81] http://www.amazon.com/THORNE-RESEARCH-AR-Encap-Capsules-Health/dp/B001124L1U/ref=sr_1_1?ie=UTF8&qid=1438831771&sr=8-1&keywords=AR+encaps

[82] No author listed. Accessed 13 May 2015 online at http://www.heartfixer.com/AMRI-Nutrigenomics.htm

[83] http://www.amazon.com/THORNE-RESEARCH-AR-Encap-Capsules-Health/dp/B001124L1U/ref=sr_1_1?ie=UTF8&qid=1438831771&sr=8-1&keywords=AR+encaps

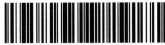

Made in the USA
Lexington, KY
30 July 2018